MW00605139

Table of Contents

Practice Test #1

Practice Questions

1. Patients with bipolar disorder are often treated with interpersonal and social rhythm therapy. This therapy helps patients
    a. recognize triggers to mood changes.
    b. manage stress.
    c. establish consistent sleep and physical activity schedules.
    d. cope with bipolar disorder.

2. When completing the patient assessment and developing the plan of care with a patient with an eating disorder, it is especially important to ask the patient about
    a. motivation to change behavior.
    b. self-injurious behavior.
    c. sexual dysfunction.
    d. goal for weight.

3. A patient who has developed sudden onset of blindness with no identifiable physical cause seems completely unconcerned about the deficit. This suggests
    a. somatization disorder.
    b. pain disorder.
    c. conversion disorder.
    d. body dysmorphic disorder.

4. An example of primary prevention is
    a. providing parenting classes for prospective parents.
    b. referring patients for treatment.
    c. conducting ongoing assessment of high-risk patients.
    d. monitoring effectiveness of treatment and services.

5. Which of the following disorders is frequently associated with sexual abuse and incest?
    a. Conduct disorder
    b. Antisocial personality disorder
    c. Bipolar disorder
    d. Borderline personality disorder

6. If utilizing sensory stimulation therapy (SST) to improve cognition in a patient with dementia, it is important to choose sensory input that is
    a. meaningful to the patient.
    b. identified through testing.
    c. easy to demonstrate.
    d. beneficial to multiple patients.

- 4 -

7. Patients who are treated with lithium to control the symptoms of bipolar disorder must be advised to avoid
   a. sun exposure.
   b. sodium in the diet
   c. dehydration.
   d. tobacco products.

8. According to Erikson's psychosocial theory and stages of development, a 30-year-old male who remains very insecure and dependent on his parents and still lives at home has probably not successfully achieved the stage of
   a. trust vs mistrust.
   b. identity vs role confusion.
   c. industry vs inferiority
   d. initiative vs guilt.

9. A patient who has had multiple arrests for driving under the influence of alcohol has agreed to begin treatment with disulfiram. Patient education should include advising the patient that
   a. drinking alcohol may result in severe illness.
   b. the patient should avoid driving.
   c. the patient may experience hallucinations.
   d. the patient must abstain from drinking for one week prior to initiating treatment.

10. A group cognitive behavioral therapy (CBT) approach that focuses on relapse prevention for substance use disorders will likely
   a. stress the importance of attending Alcoholics or Narcotics Anonymous® (AA) meetings.
   b. stress mindfulness and accepting oneself.
   c. help patients identify situations that make them vulnerable to relapse.
   d. advise patients to serve as mentors for each other.

11. If the patient is in the precontemplation stage of change regarding smoking, according to the Transtheoretical Model (TTM), the initial step in helping the patient quit smoking through a self-help program should be to
   a. advise the patient to wait until the patient is psychologically ready.
   b. advise the patient to immediately begin the self-help program.
   c. advise the patient that self-help programs are generally ineffective.
   d. help the patient progress beyond the stage of precontemplation.

12. If the psychiatric and mental health nurse overhears other staff beginning to discuss difficulties caring for an unnamed patient in the staff dining room where other staff are present, the nurse should
   a. intervene to tell staff that their comments can be overheard.
   b. reprimand the staff for violating privacy.
   c. take no action as the patient was unnamed.
   d. report the violation of privacy to a supervisor.

13. Which of the following is an example of giving a broad opening as a therapeutic communication technique?
   a. "What seemed to lead up to your panic attack?"
   b. "What would you like to discuss this morning?"
   c. "I notice that you are wringing your hands."
   d. "I understand what you are saying."

14. The four nonverbal behaviors that are associated with active listening include sitting
   a. beside patient, maintaining open posture, leaning back comfortably, and maintaining eye contact.
   b. across from patient, maintaining closed posture, leaning forward, and avoiding eye contact.
   c. across from patient, maintaining open posture, leaning forward, and maintaining eye contact.
   d. beside patient, maintaining open posture, leaning forward, and maintaining eye contact

15. Considering para-verbal communication, if a person speaks slowly and in a low-pitched monotone voice, the listener is likely to feel that the speaker is
   a. bored with the conversation.
   b. intelligent and deliberate.
   c. confused about the topic of conversation.
   d. angry about something.

16. A patient with opioid use disorder is to be maintained as an outpatient on Suboxone® (buprenorphine plus naloxone). The psychiatric and mental health nurse expects that the patient will begin with
   a. Suboxone®, with first administration 24 hours after last opioid.
   b. Subutex® for one day and then switch to Suboxone®.
   c. Suboxone®, with first administration immediately after last opioid.
   d. Subutex® (buprenorphine only) for two days and then switch to Suboxone®.

17. According to Piaget's stages of development, adjusting schemas in response to new information is a process called
   a. assimilation.
   b. accommodation.
   c. acclimation.
   d. actuation.

18. Therapy for obsessive-compulsive disorder (OCD) usually includes
   a. psychodynamic psychotherapy.
   b. flooding.
   c. meditation.
   d. exposure and response prevention (ERP).

19. If a 16-year-old female is severely anorexic, weighing 85 pounds and experiencing amenorrhea, hair loss, and cardiac abnormalities, according to Maslow's Hierarchy of Needs, which of the following needs is most dominant in this patient?
   a. Physiological
   b. Safety and security
   c. Belonging/love
   d. Self-actualization

20. A 68-year-old woman with increasing confusion is to be assessed for dementia related to Alzheimer's. Which of the following would generally preclude the use of the Mini-Mental Status Exam (MMSE) to measure cognitive impairment?
   a. Patient is highly intelligent and well educated.
   b. Patient is bilingual in English and Spanish.
   c. Patient attended school for only 5 years.
   d. Patient has Parkinson's disease.

21. When assessing a 35-year-old Arab American female, the psychiatric and mental health nurse notes that, while discussing her family, the patient uses a louder voice than while discussing other issues. This probably means that issues about her family are what?
   a. A private matter
   b. A cause for shame
   c. Of lesser importance than other issues.
   d. Of special importance

22 Which of the following ethnic groups is most likely to believe that mental illness is the result of a loss of self-control or punishment for bad behavior?
   a. Mexican Americans
   b. Japanese Americans
   c. Puerto Ricans
   d. Chinese

23. A 16-year-old male admitted to the mental health unit for alcohol use disorder has repeatedly failed to maintain sobriety and consistently missed support meetings while partying with his friends. What is the most likely reason that the patient is not compliant with treatment?
   a. Disturbance of body image
   b. Embarrassment
   c. Fear of being different from peers
   d. Guilt about illness

24. A psychiatric and mental health nurse finds herself feeling very angry toward a patient whose physical appearance and manner remind her of her abusive father. This is an example of which of the following?
   a. Countertransference
   b. Transference
   c. Displacement
   d. Projection

25. During the orientation phase of building a therapeutic relationship, the psychiatric and mental health nurse discovers that he had come to the first meeting with preconceptions about the patient. Based on this, the nurse should
    a. ask another nurse to work with the patient.
    b. apologize to the patient.
    c. spend extra time with the patient.
    d. recognize and set aside the preconceptions.

26. A patient who lost his job because of his inability to complete his work tasks yells at the psychiatric and mental health nurse that she is "mean and stupid" and ruining his life. Which ego defense mechanism is the patient using?
    a. Identification
    b. Displacement
    c. Sublimation
    d. Projection

27. Which of the following is an example of the ego defense mechanism of rationalization?
    a. Patient states she beats her child because the child needs to learn to have self-control.
    b. Patient is prejudiced against other races accuses others in the group of being bigots.
    c. Patient attends outpatient therapy to placate spouse but refuses to participate.
    d. Patient who experienced loss of a child refuses to think about or discuss the child's death.

28. A patient who has been diagnosed with bipolar disorder but has consistently refused to take medications or attend therapy, insisting that he has been misdiagnosed and has only "mild stress," is probably experiencing
    a. dissociation.
    b. resistance.
    c. denial.
    d. suppression.

29. A psychiatric and mental health nurse feels sorry for a patient because his family won't support him. The nurse offers to visit the patient's family as well as purchase some items for him. This nurse is
    a. showing empathy.
    b. violating professional boundaries.
    c. building a strong therapeutic relationship.
    d. exhibiting negligence.

30. The primary purpose of the American Nurses Credentialing Center (ANCC) is to
    a. provide political support for nurses.
    b. provide nursing education.
    c. promote the career of nursing.
    d. promote nursing excellence.

31. Which of the following is a healthy response to conflict with another person?
    a. Belief that the other person's point of view is wrong
    b. Resentment toward the other person
    c. Ability to seek compromise with the other person
    d. Feeling abandonment if others side with the other person

32. Which of the following statements could be considered a violation of professional conduct?
    a. "You look very pretty/handsome today."
    b. "Did you have a good weekend?"
    c. "I like your shoes. Are they comfortable?"
    d. "I think your comments about the patient's sexuality are inappropriate."

33. When facilitating change to incorporate evidence-based findings into patient care management, the first step is
    a. understanding.
    b. acting.
    c. deciding.
    d. believing.

34. If the psychiatric and mental health nurse delegates a task to an unlicensed assistive personnel who states she has no training in the task and doesn't feel comfortable doing it, the most appropriate response is to
    a. delegate the task to someone else.
    b. report the unlicensed personnel to a supervisor.
    c. assure the unlicensed personnel that the task is easy.
    d. tell the unlicensed personnel that you will check in frequently.

35. If a patient who has an advance directive stating specifically that the patient does not want to be resuscitated attempts suicide by hanging and is found by a family member but is nonresponsive after being cut down, the correct action is to
    a. allow patient to die.
    b. attempt to resuscitate the patient.
    c. attempt resuscitation while contacting legal counsel.
    d. ask family member for guidance regarding resuscitation.

36. The Peer-to-Peer program of the National Alliance on Mental Illness (NAMI) focuses on providing classes for
    a. family and caregivers of a children and adolescents with mental health conditions.
    b. families, partners, and friends of adults with mental illness.
    c. families, partners, and friends of military service members or veterans.
    d. adults with mental illness about mental illness.

37. If a 30-year-old patient with paranoia and schizophrenia states he does not want his parents (who are paying for his care) to visit because he believes they are "possessed by devils," the psychiatric and mental health nurse should
    a. ask the physician to intervene.
    b. allow the parents to visit.
    c. respect the patient's request.
    d. suggest the parents get a court order to allow visits.

38. Which of the following is an appropriate intervention for a nursing diagnosis of "disturbed thought processes"?
    a. Encourage patient to discuss delusions.
    b. Give detailed explanations about unit procedures.
    c. Keep a dim light on during the night to comfort the patient.
    d. Orient the patient to reality frequently and in various ways.

39. Which of the following could be an example of elder neglect?
    a. Insulting, name calling
    b. Lack of dentures
    c. Physically restraining the patient
    d. Misusing patient's financial resources

40. If a patient with severe postpartum depression admits she hates her infant but states, "I would never hurt it," the first priority should be to
    a. encourage the patient to ask for help with childcare.
    b. advise the patient's husband to monitor childcare.
    c. remove the infant from the patient's care.
    d. advise the patient to find a family member to care for the child.

41. If a psychiatric and mental health nurse is giving a series of classes about psychotropic drugs and symptom management to a group of patients with bipolar disease, this type of group would be classified as
    a. teaching.
    b. supportive therapy.
    c. self-help.
    d. task.

42. Which of the following statements by a patient indicates a readiness to learn?
    a. "I don't need to be hospitalized as there's nothing wrong with me."
    b. "It's my mother's fault I ended up here."
    c. "I already know all I need to."
    d. "I need to be in better control of my life."

43. A male patient has been following a female patient and claims that the female is "flirting" with him and using "sexual innuendos"; however, the female patient complains that the male patient is harassing and scaring her, and staff observations concur with the female patient's complaints. The male patient is most likely exhibiting
    a. introjection.
    b. projection.
    c. compensation.
    d. identification.

44. Following the death of her infant daughter, a patient suddenly started attending church and praying obsessively while neglecting her husband and other children. According to Kübler-Ross's stages of grief, the patient is probably in what stage?
    a. Denial
    b. Anger
    c. Depression
    d. Bargaining

45. An older adult with a urinary infection may exhibit
    a. confusion.
    b. hallucinations.
    c. depression.
    d. anxiety.

46. If a patient with psychosis divulges that he intends to kill his parents, healthcare providers must
    a. have the patient arrested.
    b. warn the parents.
    c. increase patient oversight.
    d. advise the patient not to make threats.

47. Which of the following divisions of the International Society of Psychiatric-Mental Health Nurses (ISPN) actively promotes the autonomy of the advanced practice nurse?
    a. Society for Education and Research in Psychiatric-Mental Health Nursing (SERPN)
    b. Association of Child and Adolescent Psychiatric Nurses (ACAPN)
    c. International Society of Psychiatric Consultation-Liaison Nurses (ISPCLN)
    d. Adult and Geropsychiatric-Mental Health Nurses (AGPN)

48. If a 27-year-old patient with narcissistic personality disorder is pregnant and has made plans to have an abortion but the psychiatric and mental health nurse is opposed to abortion for religious reasons, the nurse should
    a. discuss alternatives with the patient.
    b. provide literature about adoption.
    c. advise the patient her decision is morally wrong.
    d. support the patient's decision.

49. A psychiatric and mental health nurse has developed a successful strategy for working with a difficult patient and would like to share this strategy with other team members. The best method is likely to
    a. ask the supervisor to direct the team to use the strategy.
    b. write out the steps to the strategy and give to each team member.
    c. discuss the strategy during a team meeting.
    d. ask the physician to write the strategy as a physician order.

50. If a family member of a patient asks the psychiatric and mental health nurse what constitutes probable cause for involuntary commitment, the best response is
    a. "You should ask an attorney about that."
    b. "The person is a threat to herself or others."
    c. "The person is uncooperative with the family."
    d. "The person is no longer able to work and is homeless."

51. If a psychiatric and mental health nurse knows the employer of a patient and tells the employer that the patient is too mentally unstable to work and the patient loses his job as a result, this may constitute
    a. defamation of character.
    b. libel.
    c. invasion of privacy.
    d. battery.

52. If a patient states he feels "life is pointless," an appropriate response is
    a. "Everyone feels down at some time in his life."
    b. "Just be patient. You will feel better soon."
    c. "Why don't you try to think of some positive things in your life."
    d. "I can see you are upset. What are you feeling now?"

53. Which of the following feedback is specific and descriptive?
    a. "You were very sarcastic in the group meeting today."
    b. "Marvin became upset when you made a joke about his failure to maintain sobriety."
    c. "You tend to be thoughtless when you address other patients in the group."
    d. "You should treat others with more respect in group meetings."

54. When working with a patient with conduct disorder, limit setting includes (1) informing patient of limits, (2) explaining the consequences of noncompliance, and (3)
    a. providing feedback.
    b. stating reasons.
    c. establishing time limits
    d. stating expected behaviors.

55. In an administrative model of shared governance, the person representing the psychiatric unit is probably
    a. the department head.
    b. a team leader.
    c. any member of the nursing staff.
    d. any member of the staff.

56. Which of the following statements by a psychiatric and mental health nurse demonstrates a good understanding of peer review?
    a. "I don't mind reviewing someone as long as my review is anonymous."
    b. "My peer review is going to get him fired for incompetence!"
    c. "Peer review is a good learning experience for me and the person I'm reviewing."
    d. "The supervisor should do the peer reviews because the supervisor has more authority."

57. The primary focus of the Substance Abuse and Mental Health Services Administration (SAMHSA) is to
    a. reduce the costs associated with substance abuse and mental health.
    b. make information, services, and research about substance abuse and mental health more easily accessible.
    c. provide continuing education courses regarding substance abuse and mental health issues to healthcare providers.
    d. serve as a political action committee to promote improvements in care for those with substance abuse or mental health issues.

58. If a psychiatric and mental health nurse with many years of experience observes that a new nurse lacks essential skills, the most productive approach is to
    a. suggest the nurse take some continuing education courses.
    b. provide study materials to help improve the nurse's skills.
    c. report the nurse's lack of skills to the department head.
    d. offer to serve as a mentor for the nurse.

59. The mother of an adolescent with autism spectrum disorder with severe impairment states she is often so tired at the end of the evening that she breaks down and cries. The care support that is probably the most essential at this time is
    a. respite care.
    b. support group.
    c. volunteer visitor.
    d. spiritual support.

60. If a patient's nursing diagnosis is "risk for other-directed violence," an immediate expected outcome of intervention is that the patient will
    a. exercise control over his emotions.
    b. refrain from hurting others.
    c. express feelings in a non-threatening manner.
    d. identify methods to relieve aggressive feelings.

61. Which of the following is a Serious Reportable Event (SRE) related to patient protection?
    a. Patient is raped by a member of the staff on the hospital grounds.
    b. Patient receives an electric shock from faulty wiring.
    c. Patient dies because of a medical error.
    d. Patient cuts his wrists while hospitalized.

62. The hospital has switched to a new form of electronic health record (EHR), but the psychiatric and mental health nurse is unsure how to document patient care in this new system. The nurse should
    a. read the manual.
    b. ask for instruction.
    c. attempt to figure it out.
    d. make written notes as backup.

63. The term that relates to the belief that people's behavior should only be judged from the context of their own culture is
    a. cultural awareness.
    b. cultural competence.
    c. cultural relativism.
    d. ethnocentrism.

64. Assessment of the learner involves which of the following three determinants?
    a. Age, gender, and motivation
    b. Learning wishes, learning needs, and learning capacity
    c. Learning needs, learning capacity, and learning motivation
    d. Learning needs, readiness to learn, and learning style

65. Considering the emotional factors related to learning, high levels of anxiety may result in
    a. motivation to learn.
    b. inability to concentrate or focus on learning.
    c. lack of interest in learning.
    d. increased capacity for learning.

66. When planning an educational program for a patient with visual perceptual disorder, the psychiatric and mental health nurse must realize that the best approach to teaching the patient may be to focus on
    a. written materials, such as books and pamphlets, and pictures.
    b. audio materials, such as CDs and audiobooks.
    c. simplified materials, such as simple posters and diagrams.
    d. manipulative materials, such as equipment that can be handled.

67. When helping the family of a patient develop a crisis safety plan, which of the following approaches are appropriate to use as a de-escalation technique?
    a. Take control of the situation.
    b. Attempt to reason with the patient.
    c. Touch the person on the arm or hand to defuse his/her tension.
    d. Quietly describe any action before carrying it out.

68. A patient with schizophrenia has frequent auditory hallucinations and exhibits extremely disorganized behavior. These deficits probably result from which type of symptoms?
    a. Positive
    b. Negative
    c. Mood
    d. Cognitive

69. The usual medical treatment for obsessive-compulsive disorder is a(n)
    a. tricyclic antidepressant.
    b. SSRI.
    c. benzodiazepine.
    d. antipsychotic.

70. A patient who complains that the doctor implanted a controlling microchip in his arm and that the patient needs to cut it out is experiencing a
    a. somatic delusion.
    b. nihilistic delusion.
    c. delusion of control.
    d. delusion of persecution.

71. When developing an education plan for a group of homeless patients with alcohol use disorder, the most important information to include is probably information about
    a. community resources.
    b. inpatient facilities.
    c. personal responsibility.
    d. medications to control alcohol use disorder.

72. Which of the following is the most common reason for non-adherence to medical treatment for mental illness?
    a. Patient has double diagnosis with drug or alcohol use disorder.
    b. Patient dislikes adverse effects of medications.
    c. Patient is too confused to take medications.
    d. Patient does not believe he/she has a mental illness.

73. The most common co-morbid condition associated with schizophrenia is
    a. panic disorder.
    b. post-traumatic stress disorder.
    c. drug/alcohol use disorder.
    d. obsessive-compulsive disorder.

74. Patients who engage in injection drug use should receive immunization(s) for
    a. hepatitis C.
    b. HIV/AIDS.
    c. herpes zoster.
    d. hepatitis A and hepatitis B.

75. If the AHRQ's Rapid Estimate of Adult Literacy in Medicine (short form) (REALM-SF) shows that a patient scores at the third grade level of health literacy, the psychiatric and mental health nurse should realize that the patient
    a. will need primarily illustrated materials, videos, or audiotapes.
    b. will be able to read most written materials.
    c. will be able to read low-literacy level materials only.
    d. may have difficulty reading some educational materials.

76. The psychiatric and mental health nurse should expect that a patient with high self-efficacy would
    a. experience self-doubt.
    b. request support when needed.
    c. have low aspirations.
    d. allow others to make decisions.

77. Which of the following is an example of resilient behavior?
    a. Learning self-care.
    b. Dealing with stressful situations.
    c. Carrying out health-seeking behaviors.
    d. Having a positive outlook.

78. A Puerto Rican outpatient almost always comes late to his therapy appointments. This is probably because of
    a. lack of respect for therapist.
    b. passive-aggressive behavior.
    c. cultural ideas of time.
    d. poor time management.

79. Which of the following is an indication that a 48-year-old-patient has met the developmental tasks appropriate for this age?
    a. The patient has raised children into responsible adults.
    b. The patient has established a career.
    c. The patient has become involved in politics.
    d. The patient has a group of close friends.

80. If a patient is severely agitated when the psychiatric and mental health nurse tries to complete the psychosocial assessment, the best solution is to
    a. proceed, completing as much as possible.
    b. get all information from the patient's spouse.
    c. instruct the patient in relaxation exercises.
    d. wait until the patient is less agitated.

81. Which of the following is an example of an open-ended question that can be used when completing an assessment?
    a. "Are you experiencing hallucinations?"
    b. "Can you tell me what has been happening with you?"
    c. "Have you considered suicide?"
    d. "What medications are you taking?"

82. The psychiatric and mental health nurse notes that a patient admitted for anxiety almost constantly drums fingers on the table and taps a foot. The term for this behavior is
    a. automatisms.
    b. psychomotor retardation.
    c. waxy flexibility.
    d. nervous tics.

83. Throughout the entire psychosocial assessment, the patient maintains the same sad expression. The patient's affect would be described as
    a. restricted.
    b. flat.
    c. inappropriate.
    d. blunted.

84. If a schizophrenic patient believes that others know the thoughts in her mind, this delusional belief is called
 a. thought broadcasting.
 b. thought blocking.
 c. thought withdrawal.
 d. circumstantial thinking.

85. If the psychiatric and mental health nurse asks a patient a question and the patient wanders completely off topic in the response and never answers the questions, this is an example of
 a. loose association.
 b. word salad.
 c. flight of ideas.
 d. tangential thinking.

86. During the initial interview, the patient states repeatedly that his boss is to blame for all of the patient's problems and that the boss "is going to pay." The psychiatric and mental health nurse should respond by asking
 a. "Why do you feel that way?"
 b. "What thoughts have you had about hurting your boss?"
 c. "Can you think of other reasons for your problems?"
 d. "Do you think that this anger toward your boss is productive?"

87. When assessing a patient's orientation, the psychiatric and mental health nurse should be aware that the first thing the patient is likely to lose track of is
 a. person.
 b. place.
 c. time.
 d. current situation.

88. One method of assessing a patient's ability to concentrate is to ask the patient to
 a. give the name of the previous president.
 b. state the patient's social security number.
 c. state the patient's current location.
 d. count backward from 100 in serial 7s.

89. Which of the following suggests that a patient probably has good insight?
 a. The patient blames her husband for her problems.
 b. The patient believes changing medications will solve her problems.
 c. The patient states she is to blame for losing her job.
 d. The patient states her children purposely cry to make her punish them.

90. An example of an objective personality test is
 a. Beck Depression Inventory (BDI).
 b. sentence completion test
 c. Thematic Apperception Test (TAT).
 d. Rorschach test.

91. If a violent adult patient requires physical restraints, the patient be must be evaluated by a licensed independent practitioner within
    a. 30 minutes.
    b. one hour.
    c. two hours.
    d. four hours.

92. If a patient refuses to take prescribed medications and the psychiatric and mental health nurse threatens to place the patient in restraints and seclusion until the patient cooperates, this may be considered
    a. battery.
    b. false imprisonment.
    c. assault.
    d. malpractice.

93. If an aggressive, hostile patient has managed to remove a towel rod and is brandishing it as a weapon, the psychiatric and mental health nurse's first priority should be to
    a. disarm the patient.
    b. subdue the patient.
    c. protect self and others.
    d. leave the patient's immediate environment.

94. A patient with schizophrenia and a history of violent behavior in response to "voices" has been pacing about his room and suddenly begins shouting at the nurse, "Get away from me! Let me out of here!" Considering the 5-phase aggression cycle, the patient is most likely in the phase of
    a. crisis.
    b. recovery.
    c. triggering.
    d. escalation.

95. The concept of "intergenerational transmission" associated with family violence suggests that
    a. family violence is learned behavior acquired through exposure to violence.
    b. family violence is precipitated by genetic abnormalities.
    c. family violence almost always progresses from violence against spouse to violence against children.
    d. violent individuals tend to attack multiple generations within a family (parents, spouse, children).

96. Which of the following is an appropriate response when caring for a patient who admits to being a victim of intimate partner violence?
    a. "You should call the police."
    b. "Your partner is a thug."
    c. "I'm worried about your safety."
    d. "Don't worry. I'll take care of everything for you."

97. A 34-year-old male patient who returned from miliary service in Afghanistan has begun to have severe frightening flashbacks related to post-traumatic stress syndrome (PTSD). If the psychiatric and mental health nurse finds the patient cowering in the corner of the room in a state of panic, the best approach is to say
  a. "Give me your hand and I'll help you up."
  b. "I know you are afraid, but you are safe here."
  c. "Just deep breathe and relax."
  d. "There is nothing to be afraid of."

98. For which of the following groups may computer-assisted instruction be the most useful?
  a. Adolescents and young adults
  b. Adult males
  c. Adult females
  d. Older adults

99. A patient with borderline personality disorder was sexually abused by her father as a child and vacillates between insisting he is a kind and loving father and a horrible abusive monster. This is an example of
  a. dissociative symptoms.
  b. magical thinking.
  c. rationalization.
  d. splitting.

100. A patient with court-ordered therapy for antisocial personality disorder is very manipulative and exhibits unacceptable behavior. Part of his therapy includes limit setting. If the patient asks the psychiatric and mental health nurse a personal question, such as "Do you live with your boyfriend?" the most appropriate response is
  a. "That is none of your business."
  b. "It is not appropriate to ask me personal questions."
  c. "Why are you asking me that?"
  d. "What is the rule about these types of questions?"

101. A 62-year old-male with fragile X syndrome has been diagnosed with fragile X tremor-ataxia syndrome. The psychiatric and mental health nurse should expect the patient to exhibit
  a. tremor and ataxia only.
  b. tremor, ataxia, mood changes, paresis, dementia.
  c. tremor, ataxia, mood changes, cognitive decline, dementia.
  d. tremor, ataxia, mood changes, cognitive decline, paresis.

102. The most common behavioral therapy used to help patients with Tourette's syndrome control tics is
  a. interoceptive exposure.
  b. contingency management.
  c. massed negative practice.
  d. habit reversal training.

103. Which of the following herbal preparations should be avoided with other psychoactive drugs?
    a. Chamomile
    b. Ginseng
    c. Fennel
    d. St. John's wort

104. When screening an older adult for depression with the Geriatric Depression Scale (short form) with 15 questions, what is the minimal score that indicates possible depression?
    a. 3
    b. 6
    c. 8
    d. 10

105. The evidence-based Suicide Assessment Five-step Evaluation and Triage (SAFE-T) tool indicates that a patient has modifiable risk factors for suicide and strong protective factors, resulting in an overall low risk factor although the patient admits to thoughts of death but denies a plan or intent. The intervention that is most indicated is
    a. outpatient treatment and crisis numbers.
    b. crisis plan and crisis numbers.
    c. admission to inpatient facility and crisis plan.
    d. admission to inpatient facility with suicide precautions.

106. The patient's medication list includes both a monoamine oxidase (MAO) inhibitor (isocarboxazid), which the patient has taken for many years, and an SSRI (fluoxetine), which was recently prescribed by another doctor. The psychiatric and mental health nurse should advise the patient that this combination may result in
    a. neuroleptic malignant syndrome.
    b. hypotension.
    c. hypertensive crisis.
    d. serotonin syndrome.

107. When conducting the physical examination on a patient, the psychiatric and mental health nurse notes that the patient has dysphonia and can only speak in a hoarse whisper, a symptom that has persisted for over 6 months. Based on this observation, the cranial nerve that should be assessed is
    a. I (one).
    b. II (two).
    c. VIII (eight).
    d. X (ten).

108. A 25-year-old female with bipolar disorder is to begin treatment with lithium. Which laboratory tests should be carried out prior to beginning treatment with lithium?
    a. Thyroid function
    b. Liver function
    c. Renal function
    d. Cardiovascular function

109. When utilizing a cognitive behavioral therapy (CBT) approach with a patient who has anxiety disorder and panic attacks, the psychiatric and mental health nurse asks the patient, "What is the worst thing that can happen to you?" This technique is an example of
    a. positive reframing.
    b. decatastrophizing.
    c. thought stopping.
    d. assertiveness.

110. The treatment of choice for generalized anxiety disorder (GAD) in older adults is
    a. benzodiazepine.
    b. tricyclic antidepressants.
    c. SSRI.
    d. alpha-adrenergic agonist.

111. When assessing a patient with obsessive-compulsive disorder (OCD), which of the following behaviors would be classified as an obsession?
    a. Desire for symmetry
    b. Hoarding
    c. Repeating actions
    d. Continuously making lists

112. Which of the following SSRIs should be avoided in patients with congenital long QT syndrome (LQTS)?
    a. Fluoxetine (Prozac®)
    b. Paroxetine (Paxil®)
    c. Sertraline (Zoloft®)
    d. Citalopram (Celexa®)

113. Considering Maslow's hierarchy, in which order should the following nursing diagnoses for a patient be prioritized (first to last)?
    a. (1) Deficient fluid volume, (2) risk for self-injury, (3) sexual dysfunction, and (4) low self-esteem
    b. (1) Low self-esteem, (2) risk for self-injury, (3) low self-esteem, and (4) sexual dysfunction
    c. (1) Deficient fluid volume, (2) low self-esteem, (3) risk for self-injury, and (4) sexual dysfunction
    d. (1) Risk for self-injury, (2) deficient fluid volume, (3) sexual dysfunction, and (4) low self-esteem

114. At the end of a discussion with a patient about modifying the patient's plan of care, the psychiatric and mental health nurse states: "I understand you to say that you want to try some alternative treatments, such as imagery and relaxation, to help cope with your anxiety." This is an example of
    a. validating.
    b. summarizing.
    c. restating.
    d. assessing.

115. In milieu therapy (AKA therapeutic community), if a person exhibits inappropriate behavior, the correct response is to
    a. ignore the behavior.
    b. ask the other patients to determine consequences.
    c. help the patient examine the effect the behavior has on others.
    d. apply punishment or restrictions for the inappropriate behavior.

116. If the interdisciplinary team believes that a patient's mother may be giving him drugs during visits and wants to videotape their interactions in the patient's room, the team must
    a. get a physician's order for video monitoring.
    b. discuss it with the ethics committee.
    c. get a court order to allow use of video monitoring.
    d. have a video camera placed without the patient's awareness.

117. If a patient is being evaluated for depression and laboratory results show that the patient's free T4 level is 0.6 ng/dL (normal value 0.8 to 1.5 ng/dL) and the TSH level is 7.4 U/mL (normal value is 0.4 to 4.0 mIU/L), this suggests that depression
    a. may result from hypoparathyroidism related to pituitary dysfunction
    b. may result from hypothyroidism related to thyroid dysfunction.
    c. may result from hyperparathyroidism related to thyroid dysfunction.
    d. is likely unrelated to thyroid dysfunction.

118. An 18-year-old university student who attended an off-campus drinking party and was attacked and raped is having difficulty coping and tells the nurse, "I'm so stupid. It was my fault!! I shouldn't have gone to the party!" Which of the following is the best response?
    a. "It was a hard way to learn a lesson."
    b. "You're not to blame for someone else's actions. It's not your fault."
    c. "Yes, it was irresponsible, but you need to move forward now."
    d. "Perhaps you were both too drunk to be responsible for your actions."

119. The public health model (Caplan) of mental health care is based on the concepts of
    a. primary, secondary, and tertiary prevention.
    b. education, research, and application.
    c. patient, family, and community.
    d. community care, independence, monitoring.

120. Which of the following is an example of a situational crisis?
    a. Retirement
    b. Marriage
    c. Poverty
    d. Parenthood

121. An appropriate primary intervention for patients at risk of emotional illness resulting from trauma, such as an act of violence, is to
    a. clarify the patient's problem.
    b. refer for inpatient treatment.
    c. provide behavioral modification therapy.
    d. institute a suicide prevention plan.

122. The primary advantage of case management for community care of a patient with severe mental health issues is that case management
    a. is more cost-effective than hospitalization.
    b. eases the burdens of other care providers.
    c. relieves the patient of the responsibility to coordinate and manage care.
    d. allows insurance companies to better determine allowable coverage for services.

123. The patient that would likely derive the most benefit from Assertive Community Treatment (ACT) is a
    a. 65-year-old male with history of liver disease and severe alcohol use disorder.
    b. 40-year-old male with history of history of severe schizophrenia and alcohol use disorder.
    c. 30-year-old female recovering from injuries related to intimate-partner abuse.
    d. 20-year-old male recovering from methamphetamine use disorder.

124. A 32-year old male patient with schizophrenia has stabilized during hospitalization and has taken medications regularly and is eager for discharge but nervous, as the patient has little work history and few life management skills. The best solution may be to
    a. refer the patient to and Assertive Community Treatment (ACT) program.
    b. provide a list of community resources the patient can access.
    c. transfer the patient to a transitional living facility that provides supervision.
    d. refer the patient to a partial hospitalization program.

125. In building trust with a patient, an example of congruence is
    a. trying to disguise dislike for a patient.
    b. providing honest feedback to a patient.
    c. arriving late for a meeting with a patient.
    d. saying one thing to the patient and meaning another.

126. Exhibiting positive regard for a patient means to
    a. show the patient respect and a nonjudgmental attitude.
    b. make only positive statements to the patient.
    c. make value judgments about the patient's behavior
    d. personally like and have positive regard for the patient.

127. If a patient with antisocial behavior begins to stroke the psychiatric and mental health nurse's arm and hand suggestively during a session, which of the following is the most appropriate response?
    a. "Stop touching me this instance! You know very well that is inappropriate behavior."
    b. "If you don't stop touching me immediately, you will lose all TV privileges."
    c. "Why are you touching me? What exactly are you trying to prove?"
    d. "Remove your hand. We are discussing your plan of care, and you don't need to touch me."

128. In preparing the discharge plan for a patient and reviewing medications, which statement by the patient most suggests that more information is needed?
    a. "I'm going to work hard to give up cigarettes and alcohol."
    b. "I'm so happy to finally be getting home to my family."
    c. "Once I get home, I have to take twice as many medications."
    d. "I'm going to attend Alcoholics Anonymous meetings every day."

129. An abstract standard that a person uses to determine a personal code of conduct is a(n)
    a. belief.
    b. attitude.
    c. judgment.
    d. value.

130. Mindfulness Based Stress Reduction (MBSR) combines two modalities—mindfulness meditation and
    a. aromatherapy.
    b. yoga.
    c. massage.
    d. acupuncture.

131. Aromatherapy is used with mental health patients primarily to
    a. induce relaxation and improve sleep.
    b. increase appetite.
    c. reduce hallucinations and delusions.
    d. potentiate the effects of medications.

132. If a psychiatric and mental health nurse is creating a Johari window to gain better personal insight and the lists in quadrant 1 (open/public self) and quadrant 3 (hidden/private self) are very short, this likely indicates
    a. openness to other people.
    b. unwillingness to share personal information.
    c. limited personal insight.
    d. good personal insight.

133. If a psychiatric and mental health nurse recognizes from the expression on a patient's face that the patient is hiding something, what pattern of knowing (Carper) is the nurse exhibiting?
    a. Empirical
    b. Personal
    c. Ethical
    d. Aesthetic

134. Considering the phases of the nurse-patient relationship, during which phase is the patient likely to exhibit behavior that vacillates between dependency and independence?
    a. Orientation
    b. Identification
    c. Exploitation
    d. Termination

135. Seasonal affective disorder is most often treated with
    a. cognitive behavioral therapy.
    b. psychotherapy.
    c. exposure and response prevention (ERP).
    d. sensory stimulation therapy (light).

136. When working with an outpatient with conduct disorder who has exhibited sociopathic behavior, which of the following comments by the patient is the most cause for concern?
    a. "That pretty little daughter of your goes to Farmin School, doesn't she?"
    b. "I'll bet you have no friends outside of work."
    c. "I know more about you than you know about me."
    d. "This therapy is a complete waste of time."

137. If the psychiatric and mental health nurse is doing a self-assessment with the Nursing Boundary Index and answers "never" to 6 out of 12 questions, this suggests
    a. excellent maintenance of nurse-patient boundaries.
    b. grossly inappropriate setting of nurse-patient boundaries.
    c. inadequate setting of nurse-patient boundaries.
    d. normal, adequate setting of nurse-patient boundaries.

138. If a psychiatric and mental nurse has very negative feelings about a patient who was committed for beating his partner after the patient went off his medications for bipolar disease, the best solution for the nurse is probably to
    a. avoid the patient as much as possible.
    b. discuss the issue with a colleague.
    c. treat the patient and try to hide feelings.
    d. ask that the patient be assigned to a different nurse.

139. Which role is the psychiatric and mental health nurse assuming when the nurse assists a patient to obtain necessary services on discharge?
    a. Teacher
    b. Caregiver
    c. Advocate
    d. Parent surrogate

140. The term used to describe a patient that intentionally feigns or causes a physical or mental illness to gain attention is
    a. factitious disorder.
    b. malingering.
    c. body integrity disorder.
    d. body dysmorphic disorder.

141. The treatment for a 26-year-old female patient with bulimia nervosa sets limits regarding the patient's eating habits. Which of the following limits is counterproductive?
    a. Requiring the patient to eat in the dining room
    b. Asking the patient to keep a food diary
    c. Discussing reactions to different types of food
    d. Assigning daily "grades" for compliance with eating limits

142. A patient with phobic disorder has a nursing diagnosis of social isolation. The most appropriate outcome is that the patient will
    a. be able to function despite presence of phobic object.
    b. participate in group activities voluntarily.
    c. carry out role-related activities.
    d. acknowledge the need for social connections.

143. For patients with dissociative amnesia, the type of amnesia that involves the inability to recall a traumatic event for a few hour or few days after the event is classified as
    a. localized.
    b. selective
    c. generalized.
    d. systematized.

144. Patients with paraphilias often come into therapy as a result of
    a. desire for change.
    b. co-morbidity with serious psychiatric disorders.
    c. family pressure.
    d. criminal prosecution.

145. Patients taking lithium for bipolar disease are likely to begin to exhibit signs of toxicity if levels exceed
    a. 0.5 mEq/L.
    b. 0.8 mEq/L.
    c. 1.0 mEq/L.
    d. 1.5 mEq/L.

146. If a patient with bipolar disease takes antidepressants, they may contribute to
    a. predominance of mania.
    b. rapid-cycling.
    c. weight gain and diabetes.
    d. hypertension

147. If a patient complains of difficulty focusing attention on more than an immediate task and difficulty concentrating as well as experiencing frequent, headache, GI upset, and muscle tension, the level of anxiety would likely be classified as
    a. mild.
    b. moderate.
    c. severe.
    d. panic.

148. The Hamilton Rating Scale for Depression is intended for
    a. diagnosing depression.
    b. self-assessment of depression.
    c. determining the severity of diagnosed depression.
    d. determining suicidal ideation associated with depression.

149. The organization that provides a wide range of continuing education courses, webinars, and podcasts regarding psychiatric mental health nursing is the
    a. American Nurses Credentialing Center (ANCC).
    b. National Alliance on Mental Illness (NAMI).
    c. American Psychiatric Nurses Association (APNA).
    d. American Nurses Association (ANA).

150. A patient whose husband died in a car accident 8 months earlier is in a deep state of despair and is unable to function in normal activities. She has exaggerated expressions of anger, sadness, and guilt and often blames herself. This type of grief is
    a. prolonged.
    b. inhibited.
    c. distorted.
    d. anticipatory.

Answers and Explanations

1. C: Interpersonal and social rhythm therapy helps patients with bipolar disorder establish consistent sleep and physical activity schedules. The patients utilize a self-monitoring instrument to monitor their daily activities, including their sleep patterns. Maintaining consistent patterns of activities and sleeping at the same time and for the same duration each night help to reduce manic and depressive episodes. Patients may also engage in cognitive behavioral therapy, family therapy, and group therapy. If symptoms are severe and the patient does not respond to other treatments, electroconvulsive therapy (ECT) may be considered.

2. B: When completing the patient assessment and developing the plan of care with a patient with an eating disorder, it is especially important to ask the patient about self-injurious behavior. Patients with eating disorders often engage in superficial self-mutilating behaviors, such as cutting burning, and hair pulling, and these actions may increase as an outlet for the patient's emotional distress as the eating disorder is controlled. All patients with eating disorders should be screened for self-injurious behavior and should be monitored carefully during therapy.

3. C: Conversion disorder: Sudden onset of sensory (seeing, hearing) or motor (paralysis, weakness) deficits without identifiable physical cause. La belle indifference (unconcern) is common. Somatization disorder: Combinations of multiple physical symptoms, usually involving pain and sexual, gastrointestinal and/or pseudoneurological symptoms. Pain disorder: Pain that is unrelieved by analgesia and is affected by psychological status. Body dysmorphic disorder: Preoccupation with imagined physical defect or exaggeration of a physical defect, such as belief that one's nose is hideous, and often seeking surgical correction.

4. A: An example of primary prevention is providing parenting classes for prospective parents because the goal is to prevent issues, such as abuse and neglect, by providing education and support. Primary prevention goals are to identify high-risk populations and to intervene in order to decrease risk or to minimize negative consequences. Other examples of primary prevention include teaching mental health concepts to community members, providing education on dealing with life transitions (widowhood, marriage, adolescence, empty-nest), and educating people about the negative effects of alcohol and drugs.

5. D: Borderline personality disorder is frequently associated with a history of neglect and abuse, especially sexual abuse and incest. Studies indicate that 20 to 70% of patients with borderline personality disorder report having experienced sexual abuse, but authorities believe the percentage is higher because of patients' reluctance to admit to having been victims of sexual abuse or incest. Borderline personality disorder is characterized by fear of abandonment, unstable interpersonal relationships, poor self-image, impulsivity, suicidal ideation/self-mutilating behavior, affective instability, poor anger control, feeling of emptiness, and dissociative reactions.

6. A: If utilizing sensory stimulation therapy (SST) to improve cognition in a patient with dementia, it is important to choose sensory input that is meaningful to the patient. For example, the psychiatric and mental health nurse may show the patient family pictures and talk with the patient about the family, encouraging the patient to retrieve memories, or may

play music that the patient has previously enjoyed. Certain smells, such as perfume or food smells, may also be used to elicit memories.

7. C: Patients who are treated with lithium to control the symptoms of bipolar disorder must be advised to avoid dehydration because this may cause the blood level of lithium to increase, resulting in toxicity. Patients should drink 8 to 10 glasses of liquid (primarily water) daily and may need increased fluids during hot weather. Patients should not be on a low sodium diet but should maintain a fairly consistent level of sodium intake because lithium levels increase with lower sodium levels and decrease with higher.

8. B: According to Erikson's psychosocial theory and stages of development, a 30-year-old male who remains very insecure and dependent on his parents and still lives at home has probably not successfully achieved the stage of identity vs role confusion, which usually occurs during adolescence from age 12 to 20. The major tasks during this stage are to integrate tasks of earlier stages (developing trust, self-control, sense of purpose, and self-confidence) and to develop a strong sense of the independent self.

9. A: If a patient has agreed to begin treatment with disulfiram, the patient should be aware that drinking alcohol may result in severe illness. Patients must abstain from drinking for 12 hours before initiating treatment. Disulfiram interferes with the breakdown of acetaldehyde from ethanol, so the acetaldehyde level increases, resulting in a syndrome that can include flushing, head and neck pain, severe nausea and vomiting, third, excessive perspiration, tachycardia, hyperventilation, weakness, and blurred vision. Some people may develop more severe symptoms, such as myocardial infarction, acute heart failure, and/or respiratory depression.

10. C: A cognitive behavioral therapy (CBT) approach that focuses on relapse prevention for drug use disorders will likely help patients identify situations that make them vulnerable to relapse. Therapy may include training in behavioral skills and the use of cognitive interventions to assist them to identify triggers or situations that result in relapse as well as to provide tools they can use if faced with a situation that is placing the patient at risk, such as when associates are engaging in addictive behavior.

11. D: If the patient is in the precontemplation stage of change regarding smoking, according to the Transtheoretical Model (TTM), the initial step in helping the patient quit smoking through a self-help program should be to help the patient progress beyond the state of precontemplation with a brief intervention, which may include educating the patient and helping motivate the patient to change. Studies have shown that failure rates are high if patients attempt change from a baseline precontemplation stage (92%) with the failure rate decreasing if the patient begins at Contemplation (85%) or Preparation (75%).

12. A: If the psychiatric and mental health nurse overhears other staff beginning to discuss difficulties caring for an unnamed patient in the staff dining room where other staff is present, the nurse should intervene to tell staff that their comments can be overheard. Staff members often discuss patient care issues over lunch or breaks without considering that others may overhear. It is a violation of privacy whether or not the patient is named because some identifying information (age, gender, diagnosis) may be divulged unintentionally.

13. B: Therapeutic communication includes:
Giving a broad opening: "What would you like to discuss this morning?" This allows the patient to control the interaction and shows respect for the individual.
Establishing time sequence: "What seemed to lead up to your panic attack?" This helps to establish the relationship among different events.
Observing: "I notice that you are wringing your hands." This helps the patient to recognize behaviors.
Accepting: "I understand what you are saying." This helps to convey regard for the patient and reception for the patient's ideas.

14. C: The four nonverbal behaviors associated with active listening include:
Sit across from patient: Facing the patient directly helps to convey interest.
Maintain open posture: Keeping the arms and legs uncrossed helps to show the person is open to the other person's ideas and is less defensive than a closed position.
Lean forward: Leaning toward the patient slightly shows engagement in the interaction.
Maintain eye contact: Maintaining eye contact helps to show interest in the person; however, the psychiatric and mental health nurse should keep cultural differences in mind as direct eye contact is not the norm in all cultures

15. A: Considering para-verbal communication, if a person speaks slowly and in a low-pitched monotone voice, the listener is likely to feel that the speaker is bored with the conversation. Para-verbal communication refers to the cadence of speech (slow, fast, deliberate) as well as the tone (low-pitched, high-pitched, monotone, trembling voice) and volume (loud, quiet). Para-verbal communication often communicates the feelings of the speaker, even though that may be unintentional. For example, when people are angry, their speech tends to be louder, more high-pitched, and more rapid.

16. D: If a patient with opioid use disorder is to be maintained as an outpatient on Suboxone® (buprenorphine/naloxone), the patient will usually begin with Subutex® (buprenorphine only) for two days and then switch to Suboxone®. Subutex® is initiated when the patient begins experiencing withdrawal symptoms (≥4 hours after last narcotic dose) as the drug helps to reduce cravings and prevent withdrawal symptoms. Suboxone® contains the opioid antagonist naloxone, which may cause severe withdrawals if the patient has not been free of narcotics. If a patient takes narcotics while on Suboxone®, the patient will experience immediate withdrawal, and this provides some insurance against drug abuse.

17. B: According to Piaget's stages of development, adjusting schemas (theories about the manner in which the world functions) in response to new information is a process called accommodation. Applying the schemas to new situations is a process Piaget called assimilation. Piaget believed that there were three tasks that were essential to development and needed to be mastered during childhood: (1) how the world functions, (2) how this functioning is represented in the child's mind, and (3) how this functioning is represented in the minds of others.

18. D: Therapy for obsessive-compulsive disorder (OCD) usually includes exposure and response prevention (ERP), a specific component of cognitive behavioral therapy (CBT) designed to help patients with OCD lesson or extinguish compulsive responses. Patients rank order stressors and then, in a systematic manner, are exposed to triggers while trying not to respond with ritualistic behavior. Over time, patients should be able to face triggers

without responding, but compliance with therapy is relatively poor. Other aspects of CBT are also included in therapy, and some benefit from meditation. Psychodynamic psychotherapy does not generally help relieve OCD symptoms.

19. A: If a 16-year-old female is severely anorexic, weighing 85 pounds and experiencing amenorrhea, hair loss, and cardiac abnormalities, according to Maslow's Hierarchy of Needs, the need that dominates is physiological because the patient is literally starving herself to death. Physiological needs form the base of Maslow's hierarchy because these needs must be met first. The next level is safety and security needs followed by belonging and love needs, and esteem needs. The highest level is self-actualization.

20. C: Attending school for only 5 years generally precludes the use of the Mini-Mental Status Exam (MMSE) to assess for dementia related to Alzheimer's disease because the test is intended only for those who have at least an eighth grade education. The patient should also be fluent in English (if the test is administered in English), but being bilingual is not a problem. While patients who are highly intelligent and well educated may be tested with the MMSE, they may be able to achieve scores that are not a real reflection of their cognitive impairment.

21. D: If, when assessing a 35-year-old Arab American female, the psychiatric and mental health nurse notes that, while discussing her family, the patient uses a louder voice than while discussing other issues, this probably means that issues about her family are of special importance because speaking more loudly about important issues is characteristic of Arab Americans. People in this culture often stand close to others but avoid physical and eye contact with those of the opposite gender. However, it's important to remember what holds true in general for a culture may not hold true for an individual in the culture.

22. B: The ethnic group that is most likely to believe that mental illness is the result of a loss of self-control or punishment for bad behavior is Japanese American. Puerto Ricans often believe that mental illness results from heredity or from prolonged suffering. Chinese are more likely to believe that mental illness results from evil spirits or a lack of harmony in emotions. Mexican Americans attribute mental illness to a variety of causes, including God, spirituality, and interpersonal relationships.

23. C: A 16-year-old patient who has repeatedly failed to maintain sobriety and consistently missed support meetings while partying with his friends has most likely done so out of fear of being different from his peers. Peer relationships are especially important to adolescents who are still developing a sense of self, so if an adolescent is involved in drinking with his friends, he may be reluctant to change the dynamic by remaining sober and may feel he will be abandoned or ridiculed if his behavior changes.

24. A: If a psychiatric and mental health nurse finds herself feeling angry toward a patient whose physical appearance and manner remind her of her abusive father, this is an example of countertransference because the nurse is displacing feelings toward her father onto the patient. It's important to recognize countertransference and to examine the cause in order to increase self-awareness. In some cases, the nurse may need to discuss the issue with colleagues. Transference occurs when the patient displaces feelings for others onto the nurse.

25. D: While ideally a nurse should examine preconceptions and set them aside prior to meeting with the patient, once the nurse recognizes that his opinions may be colored by preconceptions, he should acknowledge them and set them aside so that he can establish a good working relationship with the patient. Since the patient is likely unaware of the nurse's preconceptions, apologizing is not necessary, nor is overcompensating by spending extra time with the patient.

26. B: Displacement: Expressing strong feelings generated by one person to another who is less threatening. In this case, yelling at the nurse instead of the boss who fired him. Identification: Modeling behavior or attitudes on those of another, such as entering the same profession as a mentor. Sublimation: Substituting behavior that is acceptable for one that is not, such as chewing gum instead of smoking. Projection: Unconsciously blaming unacceptable feelings/actions on someone else, such as by attacking gay people to deny homosexual attraction.

27. A: An example of the ego defense mechanism of rationalization is when a patient states that she beats her child because the child needs to learn to have self-control. The patient is trying to blame her bad behavior on the child so that she can avoid feeling guilty or acknowledging responsibility for her own behavior. Patients often try to present the rationalization in such a way that the behavior appears positive, such as by helping the child to achieve better self-control, rather than negative.

28. C: A patient who has been diagnosed with bipolar disorder but has consistently refused to take medications or attend therapy, insisting that he has been misdiagnosed and has only "mild stress" is probably experiencing denial, an ego defense mechanism. Denial occurs when a patient refuses to acknowledge a painful truth, such as a diagnosis of bipolar disorder. Denial may also include the failure to recognize the behavior or attitudes that allow problems to continue.

29. B: If a psychiatric and mental health nurse feels sorry for a patient who states his family won't support him and offers to visit the family as well as purchase some items for him, the nurse is violating professional boundaries by becoming overinvested in the patient and attempting to solve his problems for him rather than helping him to do so. Additionally, the nurse is establishing a relationship in which the patient may have unrealistic expectations of what the nurse will do, and this can lead to conflict.

30. D: The primary purpose of the American Nurses Credentialing Center (ANCC), a subsidiary of the ANA, is to provide nursing excellence and to improve health care both in the United States and internationally. The ANCC provides a number of different programs and services, including an accreditation program for nursing education, certificate programs for nurses to demonstrate expertise in various specialty areas, the Pathway to Excellence® program that recognizes organizations with a positive nursing environment, a knowledge center that provides educational materials, and the Magnet Recognition Program® that recognizes an institution's excellence in patient care.

31. C: A healthy response to conflict with another person is the ability to seek compromise and to let go of anger, disappointment, and resentment, which interfere with the healing process. Resolving conflicts is facilitated by a calm, reasonable approach that shows respect for the other individual despite the differences that serve as the basis of the conflict. The

members to the conflict should make an effort to understand the feelings associated with the opinions.

32. A: "You look very pretty/handsome today" could be considered a violation of professional conduct if the person to whom the comment is directed feels uncomfortable or if other people hear the comment and feel uncomfortable. Even though people working together often forge friendships, comments about physical appearance in the workplace are almost always inappropriate and can be easily misconstrued. Commenting on shoes is probably safe as are general questions, such as "Did you have a good weekend?" It is acceptable to directly address inappropriate comments by others.

33. D: The first step in facilitating change to incorporate evidence-based findings into patient care management is believing because unless the psychiatric and mental health nurse believes that change is possible, the nurse is defeated before beginning. The next step is to decide on a course of action, considering various options. Next is acting and carrying out the processes of change. This is followed by honestly evaluating the results and, last, acquiring understanding of the process.

34. A: If the psychiatric and mental health nurse delegates a task to an unlicensed assistive personnel who states she has no training in the task and doesn't feel comfortable doing it, the most appropriate response is to delegate the task to someone else because no unlicensed personnel should be expected to carry out tasks for which they are not trained. However, if the task is one that unlicensed assistive personnel are expected to do, the nurse should later provide or facilitate the needed training.

35. B: If a patient who has an advance directive stating specifically that the patient does not want to be resuscitated attempts suicide by hanging and is found by a family member but is nonresponsive after being cut down, the correct action is to attempt resuscitation. While people have the right to state their preference for no resuscitation, in most states this directive is not legally binding. Additionally, the do-not-resuscitate directive was never intended to facilitate suicide.

36. D: While most other programs of the National Alliance on Mental Illness (NAMI) provide classes to support family, partners, and friends of patients with mental illness or to educate mental health staff, the Peer-to-Peer program is aimed at people with mental illness. Peer-to-Peer provides 10 sessions of education about dealing with mental illness to assist those who want guidance in working toward recovery and to help people develop their own relapse prevention programs and learn to better interact with healthcare providers.

37. C: If a 30-year-old patient with paranoia and schizophrenia states he does not want his parents (who are paying for his care) to visit because he believes they are "possessed by devils," the psychiatric and mental health nurse should respect the patient's request. Patients' rights are not determined by who is paying for care but remain with the person. Unless the patient has been declared incompetent in a court proceeding and his parents granted conservatorship, the patient can deny them visitation.

38. D: The appropriate intervention for a nursing diagnosis of "disturbed thought processes" is to orient the patient to reality frequently and in various ways, such as by placing clocks within view and large signs as reminders. Explanations should be kept simple to avoid overloading the patient, and the psychiatric and mental health nurse should speak in slowly

and in a quiet voice to avoid agitating the patient. The patient should not be encouraged to discuss the delusions but should be encouraged to discuss real events or people.

39. B: Lack of dentures, hearing aids, or glasses may be examples of elder neglect, which may be intentional or unintentional. However, one cannot jump to conclusions. For example, the patient may have refused to wear dentures or may be unable to afford them. Other signs of neglect may include inadequate access to food or fluids, inadequate heating or air conditioning, unclean personal belongings/clothes, and lack of necessary medications. Insulting, name calling, physically restraining the patient, and misusing the patient's financial resources are indications of abuse.

40. C: If a patient with severe postpartum depression admits she hates her infant but states "I would never hurt it," the first priority should be to remove the infant from the patient's care because the patient has admitted hating the child and has depersonalized the child by referring to the child as "it." Additionally, a patient with severe postpartum depression is at risk for postpartum psychosis, which may further increase risk to the infant.

41. A: If a psychiatric and mental health nurse is giving a series of classes about psychotropic drugs and symptom management to a group of patients with bipolar disease, this type of group would be classified as teaching because the primary focus is on transmission of information rather than therapy, self-help measures, or specific tasks. Teaching groups usually are not open-ended but have a set number of classes at prescribed times. Teaching groups should include time for questions and answers and interactions among group members to facilitate recall.

42. D: "I need to be in better control of my life" is the statement that indicates a readiness to learn because the patient is expressing motivation. The four types of readiness to learn include (1) physical readiness (health, gender, vision, hearing), (2) emotional readiness (motivation, frame of mind, anxiety level, support system, developmental stage), (3) experiential readiness (cultural background, orientation, aspiration level, and (4) knowledge readiness (cognitive ability, learning style, learning disabilities, educational background).

43. B: If a male patient has been following a female patient and claims the female is "flirting" with him and using "sexual innuendoes" but the female patient complains that the male patient is harassing and scaring her, and staff observations concur with the female patient's complaints, then the male patient is most likely exhibiting projection, an ego defense mechanism in which the male patient is projecting his own feelings of attraction onto the female patient.

44. D: The patient is probably in the stage of bargaining, which is often characterized by increased religious practice, such as praying, as a way to "bargain" with God to help the person cope or to somehow (even magically) change the outcome. Stages include:
Stage 1: Denial
Stage 2: Anger
Stage 3: Bargaining
Stage 4: Depression
Stage 5: Acceptance

Not every patient goes through every stage, nor are the stages necessarily sequential, but most patients experiencing grief go through a number of stages, and some may become fixed at one stage, such as anger or bargaining.

45. A: An older adult with a urinary infection may exhibit confusion rather than the more typical symptoms of burning and frequency experienced by younger adults, so urinary tract infection should be suspected in an older adult who has sudden onset of confusion or sudden worsening of pre-existing dementia. Confusion is more likely to occur with severe infections that have spread to the kidneys. The confusion associated with urinary tract infection usually clears rapidly once the infection is treated.

46. B: While what a patient says is usually protected by the regulations regarding privacy and confidentiality, if a patient makes a credible threat, such as intending to kill his parents, then the healthcare provider must warn the parents of the danger under the "duty to warn" laws. These laws may vary somewhat from one state to another with some states permitting healthcare providers to use professional judgment about warning others and other states requiring mandatory reporting.

47. A: The Internal Society of Psychiatric-Mental Health Nurses (ISPN) comprises four divisions, which were originally independent organizations but came together to form the ISPN. The division that actively promotes the autonomy of advance practice nurses is the Society for Education and Research in Psychiatric-Mental Health Nursing (SERPN). Since the organizations original inception in 1983 (as the Council of Dean and Directors of Graduate Programs in Psychiatric-Mental Health Nursing), the organization has focused on graduate education in the field and evidence-based practice.

48. D: If a 27-year-old patient with narcissistic personality disorder is pregnant and has made plans to have an abortion but the psychiatric and mental health nurse is opposed to abortion for religious reasons, the nurse should support the patient's decision. The patient has the legal right to make this decision, and the nurse must use care not to impose personal religious beliefs onto the patient or try to pressure the patient into making a different decision.

49. C: If a psychiatric and mental health nurse has developed a successful strategy for working with a difficult patient and would like to share this strategy with other team members, the best method is likely to discuss the strategy during a team meeting rather than trying to impose the strategy on others without discussion. During discussion, the nurse may discover that others have also devised successful strategies and have input about strategies that are less successful.

50. B: While laws may vary slightly from one state to another in relation to involuntary commitment, generally probable cause is present if a person is a threat to herself or others (and usually the threat must be imminent). A second criterion is usually that the person is too disabled to provide self-care; however, this last criterion can be interpreted in a wide variety of ways (the reason so many mentally ill individuals are homeless and living on the streets) and is rarely utilized.

51. A: If a psychiatric and mental health nurse knows the employer of a patient and tells the employer that the patient is too mentally unstable to work and the patient loses his job as a result, this may constitute defamation of character since the information was detrimental to

the patient's reputation. Defamation of character generally involves accusations that are malicious or false. Sharing information about the patient is a breach of confidentiality. If the nurse had put the information in writing, this would represent libel as opposed to slander, which involves orally giving malicious or false information.

52. D: If a patient states he feels "life is pointless," an appropriate response is "I can see you are upset. What are you feeling now?" because this acknowledges the patient's feelings and encourages the patient to explore the cause of the feelings without rejecting or belittling the patient's expressions. Statements that may be construed as suicidal should always be taken seriously and dealt with forthrightly, such as by asking the patient if he is considering suicide.

53. B: The feedback that is specific and descriptive is "Marvin became upset when you made a joke about his failure to maintain sobriety" because it gives the essential facts. "You were very sarcastic in the group meeting today" is evaluative ("very sarcastic") without outlining the specific problem. "You tend to be thoughtless when you address other patient in the group" is too general. "You should treat others with more respect in group meetings" is giving advice ("you should") as opposed to feedback.

54. D: When working with a patient with conduct disorder, limit setting includes (1) informing patient of limits, (2) explaining the consequences of noncompliance, and (3) stating expected behaviors. Application of limit setting must be consistent and carried out by all staff members at all times. Consequences must be individualized and must have meaning for the patient so that the patient is motivated to avoid them. Negotiating a written agreement that can be referred to can prevent conflicts if the patient tries to change the limits.

55. A: In an administrative model of shared governance, the person representing the psychiatric unit is probably the department head because this model depends on the leaders of the institution. These leaders may preside over smaller councils, but they alone are represented on the primary legislative council. Councilor models may have a large number of councils that have some governance over their members. For example, each unit may have a council that sets work hours. In the congressional model, all nursing staff (or all staff) may be members of councils with varying degrees of autonomy.

56. C: The statement by a psychiatric and mental health nurse that demonstrates a good understanding of peer review is "Peer review is a good learning experience for me and the person I'm reviewing." The point of peer review is that the reviews are done by peers, those of the same rank, and not supervisors and never anonymously. The reviewer and the reviewee should discuss the review with the reviewer prompting the reviewee to seek solutions to any problems that may have been identified.

57. B: The primary focus of the Substance Abuse and Mental Health Services Administration (SAMHSA), an agency within the U.S. Department of Health and Human Services, is to make information, services, and research about substance abuse and mental health more easily accessible and to reduce the impact of these issues on communities. SAMHSA has a number of Strategic Initiatives, such as "Trauma and Justice," and "Prevention of Substance Abuse and Mental Illness," as well as advisory councils and committees.

58. D: If a psychiatric and mental health nurse with many years of experience observes that a new nurse lacks essential skills, the most productive approach is to offer to serve as a mentor for the nurse. Many new nurses lack essential skills because they have little experience to draw from and may be overwhelmed with the responsibilities of working. Mentoring is usually an ongoing process that lasts for months and even a year or more. Mentoring may be a formal or informal arrangement.

59. A: Caregiving can be exhausting, so if the mother of an adolescent with autism spectrum disorder with severe impairment is so tired that she begins crying, then she is overwhelmed and is most in need of respite care. The caregiver needs a break of even a few days in order to rest and have time for herself. If this is not possible, then part-time respite care in the home to allow the caregiver to relinquish caregiving for a few hours may help to reduce stress.

60. B: If a patient's nursing diagnosis is "risk for other-directed violence," an immediate expected outcome of intervention is that the patient will refrain from hurting others. Other outcomes that should be immediate include refraining from destroying property and demonstrating decreased acting out behavior, restlessness, fear, anxiety, and hostility. Patients may need more time and therapy to be able to exercise control over emotions, express feelings in a non-threatening manner, and identify methods to relieve aggressive feelings.

61. D: The National Quality Forum's (NQF's) Serious Reportable Events (SREs) are those events that are harmful to patients. The SREs are divided into different areas of focus. Those events that focus on Patient Protection are especially applicable to psychiatric and mental health nursing. These events include (1) discharge of a patient unable to make decisions to other than an authorized person, (2) death or serious injury related to elopement/disappearance, and (3) suicide, attempted suicide, or self-harm resulting in serious injury while hospitalized.

62. B: If the psychiatric and mental health nurse is unsure how to document patient care in the new electronic health record (EHR), then the nurse should immediately ask for instruction to ensure that the nurse is using the system correctly. Because the EHR is a legal document, information that is entered into the record generally cannot be removed, so it is essential that information be entered correctly. Additionally, in some cases, entries must be made at the time medications or treatments are administered, so instruction is critical.

63. C: Cultural relativism: The belief that people's behavior should only be judged from the context of their own culture because behavioral norms can vary widely from one culture to another. Cultural awareness: Recognizing and respecting the outward signs of cultural diversity, such as dress and physical features. Cultural competence: Recognizing one's own culture and using that understanding to avoid unduly influencing those of other cultures. Ethnocentrism: The idea that one's own cultural ideas and beliefs are superior to those of others.

64. D: Assessment of the learner involves the following three determinants:
Learning needs: Patients often disagree with others about their needs for learning, but these needs must be identified first. These needs reflect a lack of knowledge in particular areas. Readiness to learn: Physical, emotional, experiential, and knowledge readiness. Unless a patient is ready to learn or deficits are compensated, then learning may be difficult.

Learning style: right brain/left brain/whole brain, field independent/field dependent, or audio/visual/kinesthetic. Patients may respond better to teaching that matches their preferred learning styles.

65. B: Considering the emotional factors related to learning, high levels of anxiety may result in inability to concentrate or focus on learning while low levels may result in lack of interest in learning because the patient the patient doesn't perceive the need for learning. However, mild to moderate levels of anxiety are often conducive to learning because the patient recognizes a need to relieve the anxiety and may be open to new ideas to help to do so.

66. B: When planning an educational program for a patient with visual perceptual disorder (dyslexia), the psychiatric and mental health nurse must realize that the best approach to teaching the patients may be to focus on audio materials, such as CDs and audiobooks because people with a visual perceptual disorder often compensate for the difficulty reading or processing visual images by listening intently and memorizing material. Patients with visual perceptual disorder may confuse words, have difficulty seeing letters, and have difficulty understanding the overall meaning of a group of words even if able to read the individual words.

67. D: Families should be assisted to develop a crisis safety plan that includes recognizing the signs of an impending crisis and using de-escalation techniques to defuse the situation. De-escalation techniques include avoiding touching the patient without permission and quietly describing any action before carrying it out so as not to further alarm the patient. The family member should remain calm, speak quietly, listen and express concern, avoid arguing and making continuous eye contact, keep environmental stimulation low, allow the person adequate space, and offer suggestions but avoid taking control.

68. A: Patients with schizophrenia often exhibit four types of symptoms:
Positive: Includes hallucinations (auditory, visual, gustatory, tactile), delusions (persecution, grandeur, reference, control, somatic, and nihilistic), and disorganized speech and behavior.
Negative: flattening of affect, alogia (decreased fluency and content of speech), and apathy.
Mood: Inappropriate mood (excessively happy or sad) in relation to events or situations.
Cognitive: Memory deficit, impaired executive functioning, and impaired ability to interpret interpersonal cues related to communication.

69. B: The usual medical treatment for obsessive-compulsive disorder (OCD) is an SSRI because SSRIs inhibit presynaptic reuptake of serotonin. Only one tricyclic antidepressant, clomipramine (Anafranil®), has a similar action, but it has more adverse effects, so an SSRI is usually the drug of choice. Some patients also take buspirone as an antianxiety medication, and other patients, especially those with tic disorders, may benefit from the addition of antipsychotics, such as risperidone, haloperidol, or olanzapine, although not all of these drugs are not FDA-approved for OCD.

70. C: A patient who complains that the doctor implanted a controlling microchip in his arm and that the patient needs to cut it out is experiencing a delusion of control because he believes that his behavior is under the control of someone or something else. With delusions of persecution, the patient feels threatened or frightened and believes someone or something wants to harm the patient. With a somatic delusion, the patient has unrealistic

ideas about his/her body while, with a nihilistic delusion, the patient believes that an important aspect of reality (the self, the world) no longer exists.

71. A: When developing an education plan for a group of homeless patients with alcohol use disorder, the most important information to include is probably information about community resources, including shelters, food banks, free meals, free clinics, and self-help groups, such as Alcoholics Anonymous®. Inpatient care is often an unrealistic goal for homeless people with few or no financial resources unless care is mandated by the courts and covered by government programs. Patients who are homeless and addicted often have multiple problems, including dual diagnoses, which make personal responsibility difficult to achieve.

72. D: The most common reason for non-adherence to medical treatment for mental illness is that the patient believes he/she does not have a mental illness and can manage without medication. Many patients also are dependent on alcohol or drugs and may be advised to avoid alcohol or drugs with medications, so they stop the medications. Adverse effects of medications can be troubling and may cause some patients to stop taking medications. Patients may stop treatment if they are confused although confusion may also result from decreasing or stopping medication.

73. C: The most common co-morbid condition associated with schizophrenia is drug and/or alcohol use disorder, sometimes as the result of trying to self-medicate. Patients with schizophrenia also often smoke, so treatment protocols should include drug, alcohol, and smoking cessation. Drug and alcohol use disorder is frequently a factor in non-adherence to treatment plans, especially if advised alcohol or drugs should be avoided with medications. Patients with schizophrenia may also have the comorbidities of post-traumatic stress disorder, panic disorder, and obsessive-compulsive disorder, complicating treatment approaches.

74. D: According to the Centers for Disease Control and Prevention (CDC), patients who inject drugs should receive immunizations for hepatitis A and B, which are transmitted through sharing of needles contaminated with blood. There is no vaccine available for hepatitis C although patients should be screened for hepatitis C because they are at risk for the disease. There is also not any immunization for HIV/AIDS although patients may also need screening for HIV. Immunization for herpes zoster is not recommended because of injection drug use.

75. A: If the Agency for Healthcare Research and Quality's (AHRQ's) Rapid Estimate of Adult Literacy in Medicine (short form) (REALM-SF), which comprises a list of seven words the patient is asked to read, shows that a patient scores at the third grade level of health literacy, the psychiatric and mental health nurse should realize that the patient will need primarily illustrated materials, videos, or audiotapes because the patient will not be able to read most reading material, even those intended for low literacy. Assessing patient's health literacy is a critical initial element in developing an individualized educational plan.

76. B: Self-efficacy is the belief that people have control over the events in their lives and that their behavior can make a difference. Patients with high levels of self-efficacy would likely request support when needed because they have the confidence necessary to admit they are unable to do everything by themselves. Patients who lack adequate self-efficacy

often have low aspirations and experience self-doubt and anxiety because they lack faith in their own abilities and decisions.

77. D: An example of resilient behavior is having a positive outlook. Patients with resilience respond in a healthy manner to stress or adverse situations and are less likely to react to stress with anxiety while patients with low levels of resilience may react to minor stressful events with severe anxiety. Resilience is closely related to resourcefulness, which is the ability to utilize problem-solving skills, and is exemplified by learning self-care, dealing with stressful situations, and carrying out health-seeking behaviors.

78. C: A Puerto Rican outpatient almost always comes late to his therapy appointments. This is probably because of cultural ideas of time, which are more relaxed than common in the United States, where people are expected to be on time. When assigned a time for a meeting, the patient may believe that coming at "about" that time is acceptable and does not intend to be disrespectful or to display passive-aggressive behavior, and this behavior is usually not related to poor time management but rather a perception that other things, such as family concerns, are more important.

79. A: An indication that a 48-year-old patient has met the developmental tasks appropriate for this age is that the patient has raised children into responsible adults, as this is a task associated with middle adulthood (ages 45 to 65). Other developmental tasks for middle adulthood include relinquishing control of adult children, adjusting to physical changes, using leisure time creatively, valuing old friends and making new ones, being proud of accomplishments, and expressing love emotionally as well as physically.

80. D: If a patient is severely agitated when the psychiatric and mental health nurse tries to complete the psychosocial assessment, the best solution is to wait until the patient is less agitated because a patient who is agitated may not be a reliable reporter or may have difficulty focusing on the questions. In some cases, the patient may require medication prior to the assessment although some patients may be more relaxed once they feel more secure.

81. B: Open-ended questions are those that cannot be answered with a simple "yes" or "no" and don't require specific information but rather allow the respondent to answer in a number of different ways, such as with "Can you tell me what has been happening with you?" Close-ended questions, such "Are you experiencing hallucinations?" and "Have you considered suicide?" usually require a follow-up question to gather meaningful information. "What medications are you taking" is a focused close-ended question.

82. A: Automatisms: Repeated behaviors that are without purpose, such as drumming fingers on the table and tapping the foot. Psychomotor retardation: Overall slowness in movement outside of what is normal. Waxy flexibility: Maintaining positions or postures over a period of time that appear awkward or uncomfortable. Nervous tics: Rapid, repetitive involuntary movements, such as eye twitching or blinking.

83. A: If a patient maintains the same sad expression throughout the entire psychosocial assessment, the patient's affect would be described as restricted because the patient showed only one expression. A flat affect is characterized by no expression. An inappropriate affect occurs when the facial expression does not match the mood or situation. A blunted affect is one in which the individual shows little expression or in which the expressions respond slowly to mood or situation.

84. A: Thought broadcasting: The belief that one's thoughts can be heard or known by others. Thought blocking: Stopping in the middle of expressing an idea and being unable to regain the train of thought and continue and complete the statement. Thought withdrawal: The belief that one's thoughts are being taken away by someone else and that the individual cannot stop this process. Circumstantial thinking: Eventually responding to a question after providing excessive and unnecessary details.

85. D: Tangential thinking: The patient wanders completely off topic in responding to a question and never actually answers the questions. Loose association: The patient jumps haphazardly from one idea to another with no obvious association between the various thoughts expressed. Word salad: The patient uses a stream of completely unconnected words that express no meaning. Flight of ideas: The patient speaks rapidly, using many words, but ideas are fragmented and unrelated to each other.

86. B: If, during an interview the patient blames his boss for his problems and states that the boss is "going to pay," this is an implied threat. Because of the duty to warn those who might be in danger from a patient with mental health issues, the psychiatric and mental health nurse should ask directly, "What thoughts have you had about hurting your boss?" in order to assess whether there is a risk of violence. In some cases, orientation may be extended to include the current situation of the patient.

87. C: When assessing a patient's orientation, the psychiatric and mental health nurse should be aware that the first thing the patient is likely to lose track of is time, followed by place and then person. Patients may, for example, forget the day of the week or the month and date. When orientation improves, it usually does so in the reverse order, so people become oriented to person first, followed by place, and then time.

88. D: One method of assessing a patient's ability to concentrate is to ask the patient to count backward from 100 by serial 7s (100, 93, 86...). Other tests of concentration include asking the patient to spell the word world backward, state the days of the week backward, or carry out a simple three-part task (pick up the card, fold it in half, and place it on the desk). Requests that require the production of facts, such as "give the name of the previous president," are used to assess memory rather than concentration.

89. C: Good insight, the ability to understand the real situation and nature of a problem, is demonstrated when the patient states she is to blame for losing her job because she is taking responsibility and not blaming her problems on other people (children, husband) or looking for a magic solution (new medication). Patients with poor insight often look outward for reasons for problems and solutions to those problems rather than inward.

90. A: An example of an objective personality test is Beck Depression Inventory (BDI). Objective tests require the person taking the test to choose an answer, either true-false or multiple choice, and do not allow for any free expression. Other objective tests include the Minnesota Multiphasic Personality Inventory (MMPI) and the Tennessee Self-Concept Scale (TSCS). Projective tests, on the other hand, are unstructured and the responses are evaluated by the person administering the test. Projective tests include the Rorschach test, the sentence completion test, and the Thematic Apperception Test (TAT).

91. B: If a violent adult patient requires physical restraints, the patient must be evaluated by a licensed independent practitioner within one hour of having the restraints applied. The same applies for the use of seclusion. Additionally, the patient must be evaluated personally every 8 hours after the initial evaluation, and physician's orders are required every 4 hours to continue the restraints or isolation. A nurse must closely supervise the patient and document an assessment every one to two hours.

92. C: If a patient refuses to take prescribed medications and the psychiatric and mental health nurse threatens to place the patient in restraints and seclusion until the patient cooperates, this may be considered assault, which is an action that results in the patient fearing being touched or handled in an injurious or offensive manner without consent or authority. Battery occurs when harmful or injurious contact occurs. It may or may not result in actual injury. False imprisonment is keeping a patient in unjustified detention. Malpractice is a form of negligence related to professional duties.

93. C: If an aggressive, hostile patient has managed to remove a towel rod and is brandishing it as a weapon, the psychiatric and mental health nurse's first priority should be to protect self and others. Unless the nurse has had special training in dealing with patients with weapons, the nurse should not attempt to disarm or subdue the patient and should keep something between the nurse and the patient, such as a pillow or chair, and maintain a distance beyond 4 feet. The nurse should summon help and try to clear the room if other patients are present.

94. D: The patient is most likely in the phase of escalation. The 5-phase aggression cycle includes:
Triggering: Patient appears restless, irritable, pacing, tense, and exhibits increased perspiration, loud voice, and angry demeanor.
Escalation: Patient may begin yelling and swearing and making threatening gestures, exhibiting hostility and loss of self-control.
Crisis: Patient loses complete control and may begin hitting, spitting, throwing items, kicking, and screaming.
Recovery: Patient begins to relax physically and emotionally, lowering voice and acting more rationally.
Post-crisis: Patient experiences remorse and may cry or become withdrawn.

95. A: The concept of "intergenerational transmission" associated with family violence suggests that family violence is learned behavior acquired through exposure to violence, so that children who are reared in an environment in which family violence occurs are more likely than other children to either tolerate family violence as a victim or perpetrate family violence as the aggressor. Both witnessing family violence as a child and experiencing violence/abuse correlate with increased rates of violent behavior when the child reaches adulthood.

96. C: An appropriate response when caring for a patient who admits to being a victim of intimate partner violence is, "I'm worried about your safety." The nurse should avoid making disparaging remarks about the partner, such as "Your partner is a thug" because this may make the patient defensive. The nurse should also refrain from giving advice, such as "You should call the police" as this may seem coercive. The nurse must allow the patient to retain control and resist the urge to solve all the problems: "Don't worry. I'll take care of everything for you."

97. B: If the psychiatric and mental health nurse finds a patient with PTSD and flashbacks cowering in the corner of the room in a state of panic, the best approach is to say, "I know you are afraid, but you are safe here." The nurse should acknowledge the patient's fears while trying to use grounding techniques to remind the patient that he is safe. The nurse should not attempt to reach out to the patient or touch the patient without first asking for permission as this may trigger a violent response.

98. A: While increasingly people of all ages are familiar with the computer and use computers on a regular basis, the group that is likely to feel the most comfortable with computer-assisted instruction is adolescents and young adults because they very likely encountered this type of instruction in school and are likely to be more comfortable with technology and independent learning than those in other groups. The group that is the least likely to find computer-assisted instruction useful is older adults.

99. D: If a patient with borderline personality disorder vacillates between insisting that her father is a kind and loving father and a horrible abusive monster, this is an example of splitting, which is a type of defense mechanisms common to people with this disorder. The patient keeps opposing feelings separate and fails to integrate them so that the patient's emotional responses may swing quickly back and forth from one extreme to another.

100. B: If a patient with antisocial personality disorder asks the psychiatric and mental health nurse a personal question, such as "Do you live with your boyfriend?" the most appropriate response is "It is not appropriate to ask me personal questions." Consequences for inappropriate behavior should be clearly outlined, so the nurse may follow this statement with another: "If you continue to ask inappropriate questions, I will stop our discussion because that is the consequence for this behavior." The nurse should use care not to try to coax or threaten the patient into behaving more appropriately.

101. C: If a patient is diagnosed with fragile X tremor-ataxia syndrome (FXTAS), the psychiatric and mental health nurse should expect the patient to exhibit intention tremors, ataxia, mood changes (anxiety, depression), cognitive decline, and dementia. This neurological decline associated with FXTAS occurs later in life and increases with age with 17% of those between 50 and 59 exhibiting symptoms and 74% of those over 80 years. Early symptoms include difficulty writing, using utensils, and frequent falls. FXTAS rarely affects females.

102. D: The most common behavioral therapy used to help patients with Tourette's syndrome control tics is habit reversal training, which helps patients recognize habitual pattern and motor sequences associated with tics so they can identify the times and conditions under which the urge to tic occurs. People learn routines to counter the tic, such as breathing slowly with the mouth closed to control vocal tics or covering the mouth as for a cough with a tic that involves sticking out the tongue.

103. D: St. John's wort, which is used to treat mild to moderate depression, should be avoided with other psychoactive drugs. St. John's wort may increase symptoms of ADHD if patients are taking methylphenidate. St. John's wort may also increase episodes of mania in patients with bipolar disorder and may increase risk of developing mania in those with major depression. St. John's wort may trigger psychosis in some patients with schizophrenia. St. John's wort is associated with many drug interactions, including

alprazolam (Xanax®), birth control pills, phenobarbital, phenytoin, amitriptyline (Elavil®), and SSRI.

104. B: When screening an older adult for depression with the Geriatric Depression Scale, short form, (GDS-SF) with 15 questions, the minimal score that indicates possible depression is 6 (greater than 5). Patients answer "yes/no" to questions about their satisfaction with life, feelings, memory problems, and general situation with "yes" answers indicating depression. Patients who score above 5 should be further evaluated. A score above 10 almost always indicates depression. The short form requires about 5 to 7 minutes to complete. A long form with 30 questions is also available although the short form is more commonly used for screening.

105. A: Since the evidence-based SAFE-T tool indicates that the patient is at low risk for suicide because risks (such as access to guns and health concerns) are modifiable and protective factors (such as religious beliefs and social supports) are strong, the intervention that is most indicated is outpatient treatment with crisis numbers to call if the patient needs support. The SAFE-T tool has 5 steps: (1) assessment of risk factors, (2) assessment of protective factors, (3) suicide inquiry (specific questions about plans, intent, ideation), (4) assignment of risk level (low, moderate, high) and appropriate intervention, and (5) documentation and plans.

106. D: If the patient's medication list includes both a monoamine oxidase (MAO) inhibitor (isocarboxazid) and an SSRI (fluoxetine), the psychiatric and mental health nurse should advise the patient that this combination may result in serotonin syndrome, which can be life-threatening. Symptoms include confusion, hallucinations, fever, and myopathy. MAO inhibitors are no longer in common use because of multiple food and drug interactions that increase risk to patients. Patients prescribed an MAOI should always be advised to notify the prescribing physician before taking any other medication or herbal product.

107. D: Because the patient has longstanding dysphonia and can only speak in a hoarse whisper, the cranial nerve that should be assessed is cranial nerve X (ten), because it provides sensation and innervation to the larynx per the laryngeal nerves. Injury or paralysis of either or both of these nerves can result in persistent hoarseness. To assess cranial nerve X, the patient is asked to open the mouth and say "Ahh" while the nurse observes the movement of the soft palate and pharynx. Normal response is symmetrical elevation of the palate and bilateral medial movement of the pharynx with the uvula mid-center.

108. A: Before a patient begins treatment with lithium, thyroid function tests should be completed in order to ensure that hypothyroidism is not a contributing cause to the patient's depression and to serve as a baseline for subsequent monitoring of thyroid function. Lithium decreases production of thyroid hormones, so lithium-induced hypothyroidism can occur. If the baseline thyroid function tests are normal, then thyroid function is usually monitored every 6 to 12 months; but, if the TSH level is elevated, every 3 to 6 months. About 40 to 50% of patients receiving lithium develop goiter.

109. B: Asking a patient with anxiety disorder and panic attacks, "What is the worst thing that can happen to you?" is an example of decatastrophizing, in which the psychiatric and mental health nurse uses questions to help the patient view the situation more realistically. Thought stopping, forcing oneself to stop thinking about a stressor, can be used to stop

negative thoughts. Positive reframing is a technique in which the patient reframes negative thoughts, such as "I'm dying" into more positive thoughts, such as "This is just anxiety and will pass." Assertiveness training may help the patient can confidence.

110. C: The treatment of choice for generalized anxiety disorder (GAD) in older adults is an SSRI. Doses are usually started at a lower level than for younger adults as high doses may increase anxiety. In older adults, late onset GAD and panic attacks (less common) are most often associated with depression and, in some cases, physical illness, such as heart disease. As well as GAD, agoraphobia and other phobias are common conditions associated with anxiety in older adults.

111. A: When assessing a patient with obsessive-compulsive disorder (OCD), a desire for symmetry would be classified as an obsession, which is a repetitive thought process rather than an action. Obsessions commonly present with OCD include concerns about contamination, safety, and the need to act in a particular way. Some people may have persistent sexual or aggressive thoughts. Compulsions are irresistible urges to carry out certain actions, such as washing the hands, touching or tapping items, hoarding, making lists, repeatedly checking the same thing, and making lists.

112. D: The SSRI that should be avoided in patients with congenital long QT syndrome (LQTS) is citalopram because it may cause QT prolongation, and doses of the drug should be limited to no more than 40 mg/day to avoid this adverse effect. Long QT syndrome (congenital or induced), a disruption of the electrical system of the heart, is characterized by irregular cardiac rhythms because depolarization after a contraction is delayed. Patients may develop palpitations and ventricular fibrillation, which can result in death. Long QT syndrome may also result from malnutrition that leads to decreased levels of potassium or magnesium, as may occur with anorexia nervosa.

113. A: Considering Maslow's hierarchy, the order in which the nursing diagnoses for a patient should be prioritized (first to last) is:
Physiological needs: Deficient fluid volume.
Safety needs: Risk of self-injury.
Love/belonging needs: Sexual dysfunction.
Esteem needs: Low self-esteem.
Physiological needs, especially those that are critical to life, should always be a top priority. However, prioritizing does not necessarily mean that the first priority must be dealt with before the psychiatric and mental health nurse can deal with the second priority because, in reality, many diagnoses may be attended to simultaneously.

114. B: If a psychiatric nurse ends a discussion with the patient about modifying the patient's plan of care by saying, ""I understand you to say that you want to try some alternative treatments, such as imagery and relaxation, to help cope with your anxiety," this is an example of summarizing. With summarizing, it's important to accurately reflect the patient's statements without judgment. Stating the summary verbally helps to verify that the nurse's understanding is correct and helps the patient feels the patient's ideas are validated.

115. C: In milieu therapy (AKA therapeutic community), if a person exhibits inappropriate behavior, the correct response is to help the patient examine the effect the behavior has on others and to discuss more appropriate ways of behaving. With milieu therapy,

expectations are that all patients can grow and that all interactions have the potential to be therapeutic. Patients "own" their environment and behavior and must be responsible for both. Peer pressure is used to provide direct feedback, and consequences (punishment/restrictions) are to be avoided.

116. C: If the interdisciplinary team believes that a patient's mother may be giving him drugs during visits and wants to videotape their interactions in the patient's room, the team must get a court order for video monitoring because, otherwise, this is an invasion of the patient's right to privacy as well as that of the mother. State laws vary somewhat regarding video monitoring of patients, but such monitoring without a court order is usually restricted to public areas, such as hallways and nursing desks.

117. B: If a patient is being evaluated for depression and laboratory results show that the patient's free T4 level is 0.6 ng/dL (normal value 0.8 to 1.5 ng/dL) and the TSH level is 7.4 mIU/mL (normal value 0.4 to 4.0 mIU/L), this suggests that depression may result from hypoparathyroidism related to thyroid dysfunction. Typically, the TSH level rises to stimulate the thyroid to produce T4, so the levels may remain normal for a while because of the increased TSH or may begin to fall. If thyroid dysfunction were related to pituitary dysfunction, the TSH level would generally be decreased instead of elevated.

118. B: While getting drunk at a party at age 18 is likely foolish, rape is a criminal action, and the patient's getting drunk was in no way an invitation to rape. If the patient states, "I'm so stupid. It was my fault! I shouldn't have gone to the party!" the best response is "You're not to blame for someone else's actions. It's not your fault" because the patient is experiencing guilt and self-blame, common emotional responses to trauma.

119. A: The public health model (Caplan) of mental health care is based on the concepts of primary, secondary, and tertiary prevention. Primary prevention focuses on both preventive efforts for the individual and the environment to assist people to increase their ability to cope and to decrease stressors in the community. Secondary prevention involves promptly providing effective treatment for identified problems. Tertiary prevention aims to prevent complications of existing conditions and to promote rehabilitation.

120. C: Poverty is an example of a situational crisis, which is acute response to a stressor that relates to external circumstances. Other situational crises may include losing a job, environmental conditions (storms, tornados, hurricanes), and trauma (auto accident, falls). A maturational crisis, on the other hand, are experiences that are associated with different stages of growth and development, including adolescences, marriage, empty-nest situation, and retirement.

121. A: An appropriate primary intervention for patients at risk of emotional illness resulting from trauma, such as an act of violence, is to clarify the patient's problem to ensure that both the patient and the psychiatric and mental health nurse are perceiving the problem in the same manner. Other primary interventions related to trauma include focusing on a reality approach, avoiding lengthy explanations of the problem, helping the patient understand what precipitated the problem, acknowledging the patient's feelings, and showing unconditional acceptance.

122. C: The primary advantage of case management for community care of a patient with severe mental health issues is that case management relieves the patient of the

responsibility of coordinating and managing care, especially those patients with limited support systems. Patients may easily feel overwhelmed if they have to access services from a number of different resources and may fail to follow through with the care plan, resulting in recurrence or exacerbation of symptoms.

123. B: The patient that would likely derive the most benefit from Assertive Community Treatment (ACT) is a 40-year-old male with history of history of severe schizophrenia and alcohol use disorder. ACT is designed to treat patient with severe and complex multiple health problems. A case manager is part of a team of members with specialties in psychiatry, social work, nursing, vocational rehabilitation, and substance abuse with services provided 24 hours a day every day of the year in order to lesson symptoms, meet the patients' needs, lesson the families' burdens, and promote independence.

124. C: The best solution for a patient who has stabilized while hospitalized and on medication but is nervous about discharge and has little work history or life management skills because of his history of schizophrenia is to transfer the patient to a transitional living facility that provides supervision so the patient can have some assistance in managing his medications, learning to live independently, and finding a job before he has to do so on his own so that he can gain confidence in his ability to manage.

125. B: In building trust with a patient, an example of congruence is providing honest feedback to a patient because the essential element in congruence is that words and actions match and that the psychiatric and mental health nurse be honest with the patient. Incongruence occurs if the patient cannot believe or trust the nurse, such as when the nurse says one thing and acts in another way, expresses emotions at odds with words, or fails to follow through with commitments.

126. A: Exhibiting positive regard for a patient means to show the patient respect and a nonjudgmental attitude, without regard to the patient's history, behavior, or lifestyle. Positive regard develops when the psychiatric and mental health nurse makes an effort to get to know patients by spending time with them, listening to their concerns and responding honestly, and calling the patients by their names. The nurse can also show positive regard by encouraging the patients to participate in their plans of care.

127. D: If a patient with antisocial behavior begins to stroke the psychiatric and mental health nurse's arm and hand suggestively during a session, the most appropriate response is "Remove your hand. We are discussing your plan of care, and you don't need to touch me." It is imperative that the nurse maintain boundaries and respond to inappropriate behavior firmly and assertively but should avoid expressing judgment or anger. The nurse should also avoid making threats in response to the behavior.

128. C: In preparing a patient for discharge and reviewing medications and the discharge plan, the patient's statement that most suggests that more information is needed is "Once I get home, I have to take twice as many medications." If the patient will be taking more medications at home, this suggests that the patient's medication list is incomplete, a common occurrence as patients often forget medications or neglect to tell healthcare providers all of the medications they are taking.

129. D: An abstract standard that a person uses to determine a personal code of conduct is a value. Common values are honesty, cleanliness, and hard work. Beliefs, on the other hand,

are ideas that the person believes to be true, such as "UFOs are real" or "UFOs are not real." Some beliefs can be proven objectively but others cannot, and some beliefs are irrational. Attitude is the general frame of reference by which the person views the world, such as optimistic or pessimistic. Judgment is defining something as negative or positive.

130. B: Mindfulness Based Stress Reduction (MBSR) combines two modalities—mindfulness meditation and yoga. MBSR is used not only to reduce stress (its original intent) but also to reduce blood pressure, promote healing, and modify emotional reactions. Patients attend classes weekly for 8 weeks in attempt to develop a greater understanding of the connections between the body and the mind. Studies show that practicing MBSR helps to improve patients' self-esteem. The yoga portion of MBSR helps to improve physical fitness and decrease the muscle atrophy associated with disuse.

131. A: Aromatherapy is used with mental health patients primarily to induce relaxation and improve sleep. The most commonly used essential oils are lemon and lavender. Although aromatherapy is used for a number of different reasons, such as to decrease anxiety and agitation, and there is much anecdotal testimony to the positive benefits, there are few evidence-based studies to support these uses although one study showed that aromatherapy can reduce agitation in patients with Alzheimer's disease.

132. C: If a psychiatric and mental health nurse is creating a Johari window to gain better personal insight and the lists in quadrant 1 (open/public self) and quadrant 3 (hidden/private self) are very short, this likely indicates limited personal insight. The four quadrants are (1) open/public self (qualities recognized by the self and others), (2) blind/unaware self (qualities known only by others), (3) hidden/private self (qualities known only by self), and (4) Unknown (undiscovered qualities). Input is from the individual (self-assessment) and from interviews with others (public assessment).

133. B: If a psychiatric and mental health nurse recognizes from the expression on a patient's face that the patient is hiding something, the pattern of knowing (Carper) that the nurse is exhibiting is personal knowing. Four patterns include:
Empirical: Acquired from science and evidence-based research about nursing.
Personal: Acquired from experiential learning, life experiences.
Ethical: Acquired from moral/ethical knowledge of nursing.
Aesthetic: Acquired from the art of nursing.

134. C: Considering the phases of the nurse-patient relationship, the phase in which the patient is likely to exhibit behavior that vacillates between dependency and independence is the phase of exploitation. The phases of the nurse-patient relationship include the orientation phase, during which the patient conveys needs and expectations and the nurse establishes parameters, gathers information, and helps patient identify problems. The working phase of the relationship includes identification and exploitation. This is followed by the termination phase.

135. D: Seasonal affective disorder, which affects some patients when light is reduced to 10 hours daily, is most often treated with sensory stimulation therapy in the form of phototherapy in which the patient is exposed to light from light boxes that provide 10,000 lux of light in the mornings for approximately 30 minutes daily, but this duration may vary with the patient. Most patients see a reduction in depression within one to two weeks. Patients typically start therapy in October or November and stop in March or April.

136. A: When working with an outpatient with conduct disorder who has exhibited sociopathic behavior, the comments by the patient of the most cause for concern is "That pretty little daughter of yours goes to Farmin School, doesn't she?" because this could be construed as an implied threat. The patient should have no personal information about the psychiatric and mental health nurse, especially about the nurse's children. This suggests that the patient may be stalking the nurse.

137. C: If the psychiatric and mental health nurse is doing a self-assessment with the Nursing Boundary Index and answers "never" to 6 out of 12 questions, this suggests inadequate setting of nurse-patient boundaries because the nurse answered affirmatively to 6 of the questions. The three choices for affirmative responses are "rarely," "sometimes," and "often." Any answers of "sometimes" or "often" are cause for concern, and answers of "rarely" may be of concern unless the answers refer to isolated incidences.

138. B: If a psychiatric and mental nurse has very negative feelings about a patient who was committed after beating his partner when the patient went off his medications for bipolar disease, the best solution for the nurse is probably to discuss the issue with a colleague, exploring the feelings and trying to reach a resolution. It's not unusual to have negative feelings about patients, but the nurse should face these feelings honestly. If the nurse cannot provide adequate care or overcome the negative feelings, then the patient may need to be assigned to a different nurse.

139. C: The role that the psychiatric and mental health nurse is assuming when the nurse assists a patient to obtain necessary services on discharge is the role of advocate. The four primary roles of a nurse in a therapeutic relationship include:
Advocate: Informs, supports (when possible), and acts of the patient's behalf.
Caregiver: Helps the patient in problem solving and meeting psychological needs.
Teacher: Educates the patient about medicines, treatments, and aspects of care.
Parent surrogate: Assumes a parental attitude in caring for a patient as the nurturer and person in authority.

140. A: Factitious disorder: The term used to describe a patient that intentionally feigns or causes a physical or mental illness to gain attention. This disorder is AKA Munchausen syndrome or Munchausen syndrome by proxy if the patient causes the illness in another person, such as a child. Malingering: Intentionally producing the signs or symptoms of a physical or mental disorder for a purpose, such as to avoid work. Body integrity disorder: Feeling alienated from part of the body and wanting it amputated. Hypochondriasis: Being preoccupied with fear of having an illness.

141. D: If the treatment for a 26-year-old female patient with bulimia nervosa sets limits regarding the patient's eating habits, the limit that is counterproductive is assigning daily "grades" for compliance with eating limits as this may be viewed as punishment, especially if the patient's grades are low. A better approach is to use positive reinforcement when the patient does well. Other reasonable limits include requiring the patient to eat in the dining room, keep a food diary, discuss reactions to different types of food, and stay out of the bathroom for 2 hours after eating.

142. B: An appropriate outcome for a patient with a phobic disorder and a nursing diagnosis of social isolation is "Patient will participate in group activities voluntarily," as this action

would demonstrate that the patient no longer feels compelled to be isolated. The psychiatric and mental health nurse should remain supportive and honest, attending meetings with the patient if necessary to alleviate fears, teaching the patient thought stopping activities to alleviate anxiety, and providing positive reinforcement.

143. A: Dissociative amnesia:
Localized: Inability to recall a traumatic event for a few hour or few days after the event.
Selective: Inability to recall some aspects of a traumatic event for a period after the trauma.
Generalized: Inability to recall any of previous history, including identity.
Systematized: Inability to recall a specific category of information or a specific person or event.
Continuous: Inability to recall events after a specific time until the present.

144. D: Patients with paraphilias often come into therapy as the result of criminal prosecution related to the activity. Most people with paraphilias do not desire to change the behavior, and most are very secretive about the practices. Common elements of paraphilias include sexual fantasies or arousal and sexual intercourse related to non-human or non-living objects, children, or non-consenting adults. Arousal often results from suffering or humiliation of the victim. Paraphilias usually start after puberty and persist throughout life, often resulting in significant social and occupational impairment.

145. D: Patients taking lithium for bipolar disease are likely to begin to exhibit signs of toxicity if levels exceed 1.5 mEq/L. Lithium levels should remain between 0.6 to 1.4 mEq/L for adults, a narrow therapeutic range. Levels should be measured about 8 to 12 hours after the last dose because the half-life ranges from 18 to 24 hours. Sodium levels should also be monitored and maintained in normal range (135 to 145 mEq/L).

146. B: If a patient with bipolar disease takes antidepressants, they may contribute to rapid cycling, especially in patients with bipolar I disorder. Because of this, antidepressants are contraindicated for treatment of bipolar disease even though they are fairly commonly prescribed, especially if bipolar disease is misdiagnosed or treatment is instituted during a depressive phase. The FDA has not approved antidepressants as a treatment for bipolar disorder.

147. B: If a patient complains of difficulty focusing attention on more than an immediate task and difficulty concentrating as well as experiencing frequent, headache, GI upset, and muscle tension, the level of anxiety would likely be classified as moderate. Patients often function better with mild anxiety but may feel restless and complain of insomnia and hypersensitivity to noise or other distraction. With severe anxiety, patients may have difficulty completing tasks or solving problems and behavior may focus on relieving anxiety. Physical symptoms may resemble a panic attack. With panic, patients cannot think or act rationally and may experience hallucinations and delusions.

148. C: The Hamilton Rating Scale for Depression (HAM-D) is completed by the observer and is intended to determine the severity of diagnosed depression. The items on the scale are scored from 0 to 4 or 0 to 2, depending on the nature of the item. The seventeen items included for evaluation of depression include depressed mood; guilt; suicide; initial, middle, and delayed insomnia; work and interest; retardation; agitation: psychic and somatic anxiety; somatic (gastrointestinal); somatic (general); genital; hypochondriasis; insight; and

weight loss. Four other items are assessed for general information: diurnal variation, depersonalization, paranoia, and obsessional symptoms.

149. C: The organization that provides a wide range of continuing education courses, webinars, and podcasts regarding psychiatric mental health nursing is the American Psychiatric Nurses Association (APNA). Both members and non-members can browse lists of continuing education resources in the eLearning Center although some courses are restricted to APNA members. Additionally, the APNA sponsors two conferences annually. The APNA also advocates for mental health care and represents more than 9000 nurses psychiatric and mental health nurses.

150. C: Distorted grief, which results in severe despair, inability to function, exaggerated expressions of grief (anger, sadness, guilt), and self-blame, is a maladaptive grief response. Prolonged grief may persist for years with the person vacillating between anger and denial. Inhibited/Delayed grief occurs when the person is not able to get past the denial stage of grief and cannot come to emotional terms with the death. Anticipatory grief is grieving that occurs before an anticipated loss, such as when a partner is nearing death.

Practice Test #2

Practice Questions

1. An outpatient with generalized anxiety disorder (GAD) has as an emotional support animal (a cat) and wants to take the cat to work with her when she returns to her job. According to Title II and Title III of the Americans with Disabilities Act, an emotional comfort animal:
    a. does not qualify as a service animal.
    b. must be accommodated by employers as a service animal.
    c. can be certified as a service animal only if it is a dog.
    d. is certified as a service animal only on special request.

2. On physical examination, a patient with chronic alcohol use disorder exhibits ophthalmoplegia, ataxia, and confusion with stupor and somnolence. Based on these findings, the most likely cause is:
    a. vitamin C deficiency.
    b. iron deficiency.
    c. thiamine deficiency.
    d. vitamin D deficiency.

3. A patient with autism spectrum disorder level 1 cannot judge the intention behind commands, often becoming distraught over simple directions, such as "eat your lunch now," or ignoring important directions, such as "leave by the fire exit." The term for this type of deficit is:
    a. impaired social interaction.
    b. mind blindness.
    c. meltdown.
    d. stereotypy.

4. A 35-year-old, recently widowed patient was a happily married "stay-at-home mom," but has experienced severe anxiety and panic attacks since her husband's death left her with few employable skills, little money, and three children to raise. Considering Maslow's Hierarchy of Needs, the patient's primary need at this time is likely:
    a. physiological.
    b. love/belonging.
    c. esteem.
    d. safety/security.

5. The evidence-based therapy recommended for adolescents with anorexia nervosa is:
    a. family-based therapy.
    b. cognitive behavioral therapy.
    c. reality-based therapy.
    d. psychoanalysis.

6. If a therapist is basing therapy on the theory of behaviorism, the psychiatric and mental health nurse expects that the focus of the patient's care will be on:
    a. providing negative reinforcement.
    b. providing positive reinforcement.
    c. providing unconditional positive regard.
    d. assessing the patient's needs.

7. Which of the following is an example of secondary prevention for an at-risk adolescent?
    a. Refer to Alateen® if parents are alcoholics.
    b. Refer to a support group for children of divorce.
    c. Work with the patient to modify negative behavior.
    d. Provide sex-education courses.

8. A patient who has perfectionist tendencies and unrealistic expectations of himself and others is experiencing severe stress and frustration over his inability to control all aspects of his life. A useful exercise is to ask the patient to make a list of:
    a. things within his control and things outside his control.
    b. those things in his life that most stress him.
    c. things he can modify in his life to reduce stress.
    d. resources in his family and community that can assist him.

9. If the psychiatric and mental health nurse believes that the interdisciplinary team is using an unfair approach to assigning workloads to team members, the best approach is to:
    a. ask the department head to intervene.
    b. tell the team that the current approach is unfair.
    c. ask the team to discuss a different approach.
    d. attempt to modify thinking about the assignments.

10. The values clarification process has three steps: (1) choosing, (2) prizing, and (3):
    a. evaluating.
    b. assessing.
    c. demonstrating.
    d. acting.

11. You are talking to a patient who is upset. You question her about it and she simply states, "I don't understand! My daughter said that she had to leave town." An appropriate clarifying question would be:
    a. "Your daughter said she had to leave town?"
    b. "Are you confused because you don't know why she had to leave town?"
    c. "Did she say anything else about it?"
    d. "Why don't you call her and ask for more information?"

12. Long-stay inpatients may be referred to a hospital hostel program in order to:
    a. learn living skills such as cooking and cleaning.
    b. protect them from other patients.
    c. reduce the nurse-patient ratio.
    d. provide variety from usual routines.

13. One of the primary purposes of partial hospitalization is to:
    a. provide respite for family.
    b. deal with suicidal ideation.
    c. monitor the effectiveness of drugs.
    d. reduce costs of care.

14. One of the characteristics of an evolving consumer household is that the patient:
    a. receives services from multiple healthcare providers.
    b. moves from one home to another with different levels of care.
    c. doesn't have to move from one home to another.
    d. focuses on learning money management skills.

15. According to Piaget, adulthood begins when the person is able to:
    a. act independently.
    b. develop a sense of morality.
    c. see the self as distinct from others.
    d. reason systematically about abstract concepts.

16. A characteristic of an open group is that:
    a. meetings continue indefinitely.
    b. a specific number of meetings are scheduled.
    c. the same members attend each meeting.
    d. current members decide who to admit as new members.

17. The purpose of a Snoezelen room is to:
    a. teach the patient social and basic living skills.
    b. reduce anxiety and improve communication and functioning.
    c. provide positive reinforcement for patients.
    d. provide therapist-centered interventions.

18. When working with a 28-year-old female patient with bulimia nervosa, the psychiatric and mental health nurse finds a container of laxatives hidden in the patient's bed linens. The best response is to:
    a. tell the patient about finding the laxatives.
    b. reprimand the patient for having the laxatives.
    c. ignore the finding and say nothing about it.
    d. ask the psychiatrist what action to take.

19. A patient who has received long-term treatment with haloperidol as an antipsychotic agent has developed repetitive behaviors, including tongue thrusting, lip smacking, and hair pulling. The most likely cause is:
    a. pseudoparkinsonism.
    b. serotonin syndrome.
    c. neuroleptic malignant syndrome.
    d. tardive dyskinesia.

20. Which of the following is most likely to negatively impact a patient's experiential readiness to learn?
   a. A patient quit college because of financial concerns
   b. A patient has an IQ of 70
   c. A patient flunked out of high school
   d. A patient has anxiety about learning

21. If a patient with major depressive disorder is to receive an SSRI that has been associated with long QT syndrome and tachycardia characterized by *torsade de pointes,* the patient should:
   a. be advised to notify the MD if any symptoms develop.
   b. have a baseline ECG and periodic follow-up ECGs.
   c. be administered the lowest possible dose of the medication.
   d. receive a beta-blocker in addition to the medication.

22. A patient has been prescribed chlorpromazine hydrochloride for psychosis and is to continue on the oral medication after discharge. As part of educating the patient about the medication, the psychiatric and mental health nurse should advise the patient to avoid:
   a. exercise.
   b. milk products.
   c. tobacco products.
   d. sun exposure.

23. With rational emotive behavior therapy (REBT), the model suggests that (A) adversity (activating event) and (C) consequences are strongly influenced by (B):
   a. beliefs about the event.
   b. behavior associated with the event.
   c. background leading to the event.
   d. behavior of others.

24. Considering the therapeutic nurse-patient relationship (Peplau), when the psychiatric and mental health nurse encourages the patient to express feelings about an event, the role the nurse is serving in is the role of:
   a. teacher.
   b. resource person.
   c. counselor.
   d. leader.

25. A patient experiencing auditory hallucinations tells that nurse that he hears voices warning him of danger: "Don't you hear them?" The best response is:
   a. "There are no voices. You are hallucinating."
   b. "I know the voices seem real to you, but I don't hear them."
   c. "I can't make them out. What are they saying?"
   d. "Try to stay focused on what's real. There are no voices."

26. Which of the following statements by a patient is most likely to indicate suicidal ideation and risk for suicide?
    a. "My children would be better off without me."
    b. "I can't stop crying when I think about my mother's death."
    c. "My brother thinks he is so much better than I am."
    d. "Sometimes, I think this therapy is totally pointless."

27. With a patient with schizophrenia and a nursing diagnosis of impaired verbal communication, a technique used to show empathy and encourage communication is:
    a. translating words into feelings.
    b. making observations.
    c. presenting reality.
    d. verbalizing the implied.

28. A patient believes that messages are being sent to her in newspapers, magazines, radio, and television and that she must decipher them. This type of delusion is a:
    a. delusion of persecution.
    b. delusion of control.
    c. delusion of reference.
    d. delusion of grandeur.

29. A patient repeats the same word over and over, "cake," when asked if he'd like dessert. This is an example of:
    a. associative looseness.
    b. perseveration.
    c. tangentiality.
    d. echolalia.

30. The most common type of hallucination experienced by psychiatric patients is:
    a. auditory.
    b. visual.
    c. tactile.
    d. olfactory.

31. A patient becomes overwhelmed when asked to make even a simple decision, such as choosing between an egg and toast or cereal for breakfast. This probably results from:
    a. depersonalization.
    b. anhedonia.
    c. regression.
    d. emotional ambivalence.

32. An appropriate nursing diagnosis for a patient who experiences delusional thinking, decreased volition, impaired problem solving, impaired abstract thinking, and suspicion of others is:
    a. disturbed sensory perception.
    b. social isolation.
    c. disturbed thought processes.
    d. self-care deficit.

33. A patient who looks at a picture of red roses and perceives a monster dripping blood from its mouth is experiencing:
    a. an illusion.
    b. a delusion.
    c. a hallucination.
    d. magical thinking.

34. A patient may utilize the ego defense mechanism of *sublimation* in order to:
    a. voluntarily block unpleasant emotions.
    b. negate an intolerable experience.
    c. retreat to an earlier stage of development.
    d. redirect socially unacceptable impulses.

35. A patient whose partner has left him for someone else and who spends an hour discussing all of the positive aspects of being single is probably utilizing the ego defense mechanism of:
    a. displacement.
    b. intellectualism.
    c. denial.
    d. rationalization.

36. The psychiatric and mental health nurse is teaching an unmotivated patient about managing her disorder and medications. The best approach is probably to:
    a. provide short lessons and assignments.
    b. use illustrated materials only.
    c. institute a reward/punishment system.
    d. provide independent study materials.

37. Which of the following statements/questions by the psychiatric and mental health nurse indicates that the nurse is fulfilling the role of resource person?
    a. "You must attend group therapy every day after lunch."
    b. "Take this medication in the morning so it doesn't interfere with sleep."
    c. "Let me show you around and answer any questions you might have."
    d. "How do you feel about what your father said about you?"

38. According to Peplau's Interpersonal Theory, a patient who is miserly, suspicious, and envious of others has likely failed to complete developmental tasks associated with the stage of:
    a. infancy (learning to count on others).
    b. toddlerhood (learning to delay satisfaction).
    c. early childhood (identifying oneself).
    d. late childhood (developing participatory skills).

39. Which of the following is a characteristic of crises?
    a. The precipitating event may be unidentifiable.
    b. Most individuals never experience a crisis.
    c. Crises may be acute or chronic.
    d. Crises are personal in nature.

40. When creating an environment conducive to learning for one-on-one instruction for a patient with anxiety disorder, the best environment is:
    a. brightly-lit, quiet, and uncluttered.
    b. dimly lit, quiet, and uncluttered.
    c. patient's preference.
    d. secluded from others and quiet.

41. The type of exercise that may reduce symptoms of anxiety and depression is:
    a. aerobic.
    b. isometric.
    c. stretching.
    d. weight lifting.

42. Which of the following is prohibited by Health Insurance Portability and Accountability Act (HIPAA) regulations?
    a. Using a unique identifier and password to access the patient's electronic health record.
    b. Informing the parents of a 16-year-old patient about a change in the patient's condition.
    c. Providing laboratory results to a patient upon the patient's request.
    d. Allowing another nurse not assigned to the patient to read the patient's records.

43. A patient is able to read printed directions out loud with minimal difficulty. In order to test for comprehension, the psychiatric and mental health nurse should:
    a. give the patient an immediate quiz about the content.
    b. ask the patient to paraphrase the directions.
    c. complete a reading assessment.
    d. give the patient a quiz about the content in 2 days.

44. The psychiatric and mental health nurse is conducting a smoking cessation class for a group of patients, and two patients are adamant that they plan to resume smoking after discharge from the psychiatric facility. The best solution is to:
    a. exclude the two patients from the group.
    b. warn the patients that smoking could endanger their lives.
    c. arrange for the two patients to meet a person with lung cancer from smoking.
    d. provide information about symptoms of concern, such as increased cough.

45. A 42-year-old homeless woman with substance abuse disorder related to long-term heroin use has been admitted on a 72-hour hold after assaulting another homeless person and is about to be discharged. Which of the following outpatient resources is the priority?
    a. Narcotics Anonymous®
    b. A group therapy program
    c. A methadone program
    d. A home health agency

46. Screening for intimate partner abuse should be done for all female patients:
    a. age 12 or older.
    b. age 14 or older.
    c. age 16 or older.
    d. age 18 or older.

47. Which of the following behaviors would differentiate aggression from anger?
    a. Passive-aggressive behavior
    b. Holding clenched fists
    c. Yelling and shouting
    d. Verbal threats

48. The best tool to ensure medication adherence is:
    a. a system of rewards/consequences.
    b. free medications.
    c. patient education.
    d. automated message reminders.

49. Under provisions of the Americans with Disabilities Act (ADA) related to people with psychiatric disabilities, employers are required to:
    a. provide reasonable accommodations.
    b. hire a person with psychiatric disabilities.
    c. provide any work accommodations that the person requests.
    d. hold the person's position indefinitely until the person can return to work.

50. A realistic goal for relapse prevention therapy (RPT) is to:
    a. prevent all relapses.
    b. emphasize the negative aspects of relapse.
    c. end the patient's association with previous friends.
    d. help patients deal with the potential for relapse.

51. In order for a patient with a terminal disease to be admitted to a hospice program under Medicare, the physician must certify that the patient's death is expected within:
    a. one month.
    b. 6 months.
    c. 8 months.
    d.12 months.

52. If a patient who has been using heroin is admitted to the psychiatric unit, how long after the last dose was taken is the patient likely to exhibit withdrawal symptoms?
    a. 6 to 12 hours
    b. 12 to 24 hours
    c. 24 to 48 hours
    d. 48 to 74 hours

53. The primary reason that milieu therapy (therapeutic community) is less frequently used as a therapeutic approach currently is that:
    a. it was ineffective for the majority of patients.
    b. it required expensive and time-consuming training.
    c. the length of stay in psychiatric units has decreased.
    d. hospitals often had insufficient space to accommodate the programs.

54. A patient has difficulty with both verbal and nonverbal communication that is appropriate for the social context, is unable to match communication to the needs of the listener, and has difficulty recognizing clues for turn-taking but exhibits no repetitive motor movements, fixated interests, or abnormal response to sensory input. These signs and symptoms are characteristic of:
a. autism spectrum disorder, level 1.
b. autism spectrum disorder, level 2.
c. autism spectrum disorder, level 3.
d. social (pragmatic) communication disorder.

55. Which of the following are the primary components of dialectical behavioral therapy (DBT) used to treat borderline personality disorder?
a. Psychotherapy and group therapy
b. Meditation and psychoanalysis
c. Meditation and group therapy
d. Group therapy and psychoanalysis

56. A patient with antisocial personality disorder tells the psychiatric and mental health nurse (who is sensitive about her weight) that other staff members are making fun of her appearance and state she is "fat and lazy." The nurse should:
a. confront staff members.
b. report this to the department head.
c. advise the patient that he is lying.
d. advise the patient that his comments are inappropriate.

57. A 22-year-old patient was diagnosed with major depressive disorder after 6 months of depression but did not respond to a trial of an SSRI or another trial of an SNRI. The most likely next step is to:
a. change to a tricyclic antidepressant.
b. explore the possible diagnosis of bipolar disorder.
c. try a different SSRI.
d. consider electroconvulsive therapy (ECT).

58. The dissociative subtype of post-traumatic stress disorder (PTSD) is characterized by:
a. hallucinations and delusions.
b. aggression and depression.
c. depersonalization and derealization.
d. depression and panic attacks.

59. Which of the following statements by a patient in cognitive behavioral therapy for major depressive disorder suggests that the patient, who is experiencing negative thoughts, is applying principles learned in therapy?
a. "I know I need to change because I feel so worthless all the time."
b. "I can't fix this situation, so I'm going to think about taking a vacation."
c. "I should have known better than to think I could fix this situation."
d. "I want to feel better about this situation."

60. Interpersonal therapy is generally most effective for:
   a. depressive episodes associated with specific situations.
   b. major depressive episodes.
   c. depressive episodes associated with bipolar disorder.
   d. depressive episodes associated with PTSD.

61. Which of the following is an example of self-harm?
   a. A patient engages in body piercing
   b. A patient tells herself that she is a failure
   c. A patient cuts herself on the legs with a razor
   d. A patient attempts suicide by cutting her wrists

62. According to Erikson's stages of human development, the key event for people between the ages of 40 to 65 years (generativity vs. stagnation) is:
   a. independence.
   b. love relationships.
   c. reflection/acceptance of one's life.
   d. parenting.

63. If a psychiatric and mental health nurse is physically attacked by a patient and the nurse suffers a broken arm as a result, this would be a Serious Reportable Event (SRE) in the category of:
   a. care management event.
   b. patient protection event.
   c. environmental event.
   d. potential criminal event.

64. For a patient taking lithium to control bipolar disorder, the serum level for maintenance should be:
   a. 0.5 to 1.5 mEq/L.
   b. 1.5 to 2.0 mEq/L.
   c. 2 to 3 mEq/L.
   d. 3 to 4 mEq/L.

65. Which of the following is a common myth associated with suicide?
   a. Once a suicide risk, not always a suicide risk.
   b. People who talk about suicide often attempt suicide.
   c. People who commit suicide always do so to hurt only themselves.
   d. There are many ways to help people who are suicidal.

66. If a patient expresses lack of control over her life and personal situation and doesn't participate in her own care or decision-making, an appropriate nursing diagnosis is:
   a. risk for injury.
   b. powerlessness.
   c. low self-esteem.
   d. ineffective coping.

67. If, while conducting a peer review, the psychiatric and mental health nurse observes the other nurse using non-therapeutic communication techniques with a patient, the best response is to:
    a. immediately intervene.
    b. discuss at a post-review meeting.
    c. report the observation to a supervisor.
    d. ignore it as it does not constitute negligence.

68. If a patient has an intellectual disability and an IQ of 45, a realistic maximal expectation is that the patient:
    a. may develop minimal self-help skills.
    b. may be able to acquire vocational skills.
    c. may be capable of working in a sheltered workshop.
    d. may benefit from systematic habit training.

69. According to the American Nurses Association *Code of Ethics,* who is responsible for the psychiatric and mental health nurse's nursing practice when employed in a hospital?
    a. The hospital
    b. The nursing director
    c. The department head
    d. The individual nurse

70. If a patient's family caregivers are interested in taking classes or training to better help them assist the patient and to cope more effectively with the patient's illness, the most appropriate referral is to the:
    a. National Alliance on Mental Illness (NAMI).
    b. Substance Abuse and Mental Health Services Administration (SAMHSA).
    c. American Psychiatric Nurses Association (APNA).
    d. National Institute of Mental Health (NIMH).

71. If a psychiatric and mental health nurse has agreed to formally mentor a newly-graduated registered nurse for a 2-year period, how frequently should the mentor plan to meet with the mentee during the first year?
    a. Daily
    b. Monthly
    c. Weekly
    d. On request

72. A Southeast Asian patient is admitted to the psychiatric unit with major depressive episode. On physical examination, the psychiatric nurse notes a symmetrical pattern of bruising and petechiae up and down the back, chest, and shoulders, and across the forehead. This probably indicates:
    a. coining.
    b. cupping.
    c. a sadistic/masochistic ritual.
    d. physical abuse.

73. Which of the following may be a warning sign that a psychiatric and mental health nurse has breached professional patient-nurse boundaries?
     a. Spending extra time with a patient in crisis
     b. Acknowledging personal preferences for some types of patients
     c. Confiding to a patient that the nurse is having financial problems
     d. Thinking outside of work about better ways to meet a patient's needs

74. When a psychiatric and mental health nurse says to a patient, "Tell me about how you were sexually abused by your father," this is an example of the non-therapeutic communication technique of:
     a. interpreting.
     b. requesting an example.
     c. approving/disapproving.
     d. probing.

75. Which of the following is an example of feedback that is directed at an action that the patient cannot modify?
     a. "Your comment is inappropriate."
     b. "You seem angry at your therapist."
     c. "You have memory problems because of your alcohol abuse."
     d. "I noticed that you didn't make eye contact with your son."

76. The emphasis of reality therapy (Glasser) is on:
     a. the present and personal responsibility.
     b. past behavior and causes.
     c. labeling behavior and symptoms.
     d. stress reduction techniques.

77. Considering assertiveness training, an example of "clouding/fogging" in response to the statement, "You should be fired for the way you handled that situation," is:
     a. "You're right. I could have handled that situation better."
     b. "Of course you're right. We all know you are always right."
     c. "What exactly did I do wrong?"
     d. "I can see you're upset. Let's discuss this later."

78. According to cognitive behavioral therapy (CBT), the type of automatic thought exemplified when a patient states, "My mother thinks I'm a failure," is:
     a. personalizing.
     b. all-or-nothing.
     c. discounting positives.
     d. mind reading.

79. The most appropriate tool to differentiate delirium from other types of confusion is the:
     a. Mini-Mental State Exam.
     b. Confusion Assessment Method.
     c. Mini-cog.
     d. Time and Change Test.

80. If a patient with substance abuse disorder states he has been using "beanies," the psychiatric and mental health nurse should understand that the patient is referring to:
    a. marijuana.
    b. cocaine.
    c. methamphetamine.
    d. heroin.

81. Which of the following tasks for a patient is one that is appropriate for a psychiatric and mental health nurse to delegate to unlicensed assistive personnel?
    a. Applying restraints
    b. Taking routine vital signs
    c. Performing a psychosocial assessment
    d. Conducting health teaching

82. A patient who has been very upset because his girlfriend broke up with him when he was hospitalized begins to follow the psychiatric and mental health nurse, insulting her and suggesting that she is trying to undermine his therapy. This is likely an example of:
    a. countertransference.
    b. transference.
    c. obsession.
    d. displacement.

83. In a group process, the three major types of roles that group members assume within the group are (1) completing group tasks, (2) supporting the group process, and (3):
    a. fulfilling personal needs.
    b. controlling the group.
    c. challenging the group.
    d. providing moral guidance.

84. The most appropriate intervention for severe confusion and agitation in a patient with neurocognitive disorder due to Alzheimer's disease is:
    a. an SSRI.
    b. an antipsychotic.
    c. an anticonvulsant.
    d. non-pharmacological measures.

85. Which of the following is a characteristic of binge-eating disorder (BED)?
    a. Eating more slowly than usual
    b. Eating alone out of embarrassment at the amount of food eaten
    c. Eating large amounts of food in response to hunger
    d. Eating large amounts but never feeling full

86. If a patient has a nursing diagnosis of social isolation, which of the descriptions is appropriate to document in the patient's electronic health record (EHR)?
    a. "Patient exhibiting social isolation and lack of cooperation with group activities."
    b. "Patient increasingly withdrawn and uncooperative with therapy."
    c. "Patient stays alone in room, stating 'Go away,' when asked to participate in group activities."
    d. "Patient isolating himself and being increasingly unfriendly and resistive to group activities."

87. The four essential components of informed consent before a patient can make a decision about care are:
    a. competence, disclosure, options, and voluntarism.
    b. competence, comprehension, non-coercion, and disclosure.
    c. voluntarism, competence, non-coercion, and disclosure.
    d. voluntarism, competence, disclosure, and comprehension.

88. Which of the following organizations/agencies provides the Evidence-Based Practices (EBP) Web Guide for treatment of mental and substance abuse disorders?
    a. Substance Abuse and Mental Health Services Administration (SAMHSA)
    b. United States Food and Drug Administration (FDA)
    c. National Alliance on Mental Illness (NAMI)
    d. American Psychological Association (APA)

89. If a patient with substance abuse disorder has a nursing diagnosis of *ineffective coping* in the nursing care plan, an appropriate expected outcome would be:
    a. Patient makes positive choices
    b. Patient begins to recognize maladaptive behaviors
    c. Patient does not act on impulses
    d. Patient verbalizes feelings

90. According to Maslow's Hierarchy of Needs, which of the following nursing diagnoses would have priority?
    a. Risk for injury
    b. Ineffective coping
    c. Sleep deprivation
    d. Social isolation

91. According to the four phases of alcoholic drinking behavior (Jellinek), blackouts are a characteristic of:
    a. Phase I, Pre-alcoholic.
    b. Phase II, Early Alcoholic.
    c. Phase III, Crucial.
    d. Phase IV, Chronic.

92. Typical behavior associated with intoxication from inhalant use includes:
    a. euphoria, lethargy, impaired judgment, and slurred speech.
    b. belligerence, assaultiveness, impaired judgment, and slurred speech.
    c. restlessness, nervousness, insomnia, and flushed face.
    d. euphoria, anxiety, suspicion, and sensation of slow passage of time.

93. Which of the following are examples of negative symptoms associated with schizophrenia?
    a. Hallucinations and delusions
    b. Inappropriate clothing, aggressive behavior, stereotyped behavior
    c. Abnormal though processes and speech patterns
    d. Blunt or flat affect, avolition, and reduced speech

94. With obsessive-compulsive disorder, which of the following is a common compulsion?
   a. Experiencing unwanted sexually aggressive thoughts
   b. Being fearful of committing a sin
   c. Repeatedly checking to make sure the door is locked
   d. Experiencing constant fear and concerns about safety

95. A patient with schizophrenia with catatonia has sat in the same chair with the right arm extended for an hour after the phlebotomist extended the arm for a blood draw. This is an example of:
   a. posturing.
   b. waxy flexibility.
   c. anergia.
   d. mimicry.

96. When conducting an outreach program to screen homeless people for mental health and/or substance abuse disorders, the best method to use to encourage participation is to:
   a. offer free food, water, and hygiene products.
   b. advertise on TV and radio and in local newspapers.
   c. ask the police department to refer homeless people.
   d. advertise through community volunteers.

97. Regular membership in the American Psychiatric Nurses Association (APNA) is available to:
   a. international nurses as well as those working in the United States.
   b. all licensed registered nurses.
   c. all nurses with baccalaureate or master's degrees.
   d. all mental health professionals.

98. The most commonly cited barrier to psychiatric treatment for mental health patients at all levels of severity is:
   a. social stigma.
   b. financial costs.
   c. low perceived need.
   d. access.

99. If a patient who was voluntarily committed to a psychiatric facility wants to leave and is restrained from doing so by a psychiatric and mental health nurse, this may constitute:
   a. assault and battery.
   b. intentional tort.
   c. negligence.
   d. false imprisonment.

100. A patient with schizophrenia is admitted to the hospital after developing polydipsia, drinking water excessively and becoming increasing confused and psychotic. The electrolyte imbalance of most concern is:
   a. hyponatremia.
   b. hypernatremia.
   c. hypocalcemia.
   d. hypercalcemia.

101. According to Havighurst's theory of adult development, middle age is characterized by:
    a. Managing a home and finding a congenial social group.
    b. Establishing ties with those in the same age group and adjusting to a decrease in physical strength.
    c. Establishing physical living arrangements that are satisfactory.
    d. Achieving civil/social responsibility and maintaining an economic standard of living.

102. The medication used to control cocaine craving during withdrawal is:
    a. Naloxone.
    b. Bromocriptine.
    c. Lorazepam.
    d. Sodium bicarbonate.

103. Which theory states that a change in one family member's behavior will affect others in the family?
    a. Health belief model (Rosenstock)
    b. Theory of planned behavior (Azjen)
    c. Family systems theory (Bowen)
    d. Theory of reasoned action (Fishbein and Azjen)

104. What is a good strategy for helping an elderly client overcome feelings of low self-esteem related to chronic illness and loss of autonomy?
    a. Praise the client constantly for any activities.
    b. Tell the client she has no reason to feel so depressed.
    c. Provide opportunities for the client to make decisions.
    d. Encourage the patient to focus on positive factors.

105. A 27-year-old male with a history of drug and alcohol abuse, stealing, and bullying behavior has been working with the psychiatric/mental health nurse on educational issues related to substance abuse, self-esteem, and anger. The primary determinants of the effectiveness of education are:
    a. Observed behavior modification and compliance.
    b. Self-reported behavior modification and compliance.
    c. Positive reports from the probation officer.
    d. Drug and alcohol abstinence verified by testing.

106. A 30-year-old woman with a history of bulimia nervosa (BN) since adolescence is receiving therapy to help her want to change, accept responsibility for change, and remain committed to change. The patient is guided through different stages, beginning with precontemplation. This type of therapy is referred to as:
    a. Cognitive behavioral therapy (CBT).
    b. Motivation enhancement therapy.
    c. Interpersonal psychotherapy.
    d. Family therapy.

107. Which of the following disorders is characterized by personality disintegration and distortion in the perception of reality, thought processes, and social development?
    a. Depression.
    b. Bipolar disorder.
    c. Schizophrenia.
    d. Narcissistic personality disorder.

108. Which of the following best describes Kolb's model of experiential learning?
    a. Knowledge develops from experience interacting with cognition and perception.
    b. Knowledge and experience are equally important.
    c. Experience precedes knowledge in learning.
    d. Learning cannot be acquired without experience and perception.

109. In Piaget's theory of cognitive development, the stage in which the child or adolescent has a better understanding of cause and effect and a good ability to understand concrete objects and the concept of conservation is:
    a. Concrete operational.
    b. Preoperational.
    c. Sensorimotor.
    d. Formal operational.

110. A 45-year-old male is married with two children. He lost his job 6 months ago and has been unable to make house payments. He has become increasingly temperamental, has explosive outbursts of anger, and attacked his wife during an argument, hitting her in the face and throwing her against the wall. The type of emotional crisis he is likely experiencing is:
    a. Adventitious/Social.
    b. Situational/Dispositional.
    c. Maturational/Developmental.
    d. Psychopathological.

111. The theory that outlines nine personality parameters to explain how children respond to events and describes the difficult child, the child who is slow to warm up to new people and circumstances, and the child who is easy to manage and adaptable is:
    a. Resilience theory.
    b. Social learning theory (Bandura).
    c. Temperament theory (Chase and Thomas).
    d. Theory of moral development (Kohlberg).

112. A parent stops the psychiatric/mental health nurse and states, "Could you tell me what is wrong with the patient across the hall from my son? He seems so agitated." The response that complies with the Health Insurance Portability and Accountability Act (HIPAA) is:
    a. "The law doesn't allow me to give out any information about patients in order to protect their privacy and safety."
    b. "His mother is in the lounge. You can go ask her."
    c. "Why are you asking?"
    d. "He has bipolar disease, like your son."

113. An 8-year-old boy has been sleeping poorly, complaining of stomachaches, crying frequently, and refusing to go to school. A complete physical examination ruled out a physical ailment. As part of an assessment for anxiety, the simplest assessment tool to use with a child is the:
   a. Hamilton Anxiety Scale (HAS). [MORE COMMON ACRONYM APPEARS TO BE "HAMA"]
   b. Beck Anxiety Inventory (BAI).
   c. Beck Depression Inventory (BDI).
   d. Revised Children's Manifest Anxiety Scale (RCMAS).

114. A 16-year-old girl is being treated with fluoxetine and cognitive behavioral therapy (CBT) for severe anxiety and depression 6 months after the death of her mother. The girl must be monitored and regularly assessed for:
   a. Substance abuse.
   b. Polypharmacy.
   c. Suicidal ideation.
   d. Noncompliance.

115. A prevention strategy that encourages physicians, nurses, and other healthcare providers to discuss substance abuse with all adolescents is an example of:
   a. Secondary prevention.
   b. Universal primary prevention.
   c. Indicated primary prevention.
   d. Targeted primary prevention.

116. A 76-year-old female dresses in youthful styles, acts in a girlish manner, and states repeatedly that she hates getting older. According to Erikson's psychosocial development model, which stage is she experiencing?
   a. Identity vs role confusion
   b. Industry vs. inferiority
   c. Ego integrity vs despair
   d. Generativity vs stagnation

117. Because combining monoamine oxidase inhibitors (MAOIs) with some foods may cause adverse reactions (hypertension, headache, diaphoresis, cardiac abnormalities, intracerebral hemorrhage), patients taking MAOIs should be advised to avoid the following foods/beverages:
   a. Alcohol and grapefruit juice.
   b. Alcohol, products containing caffeine (tea, cola, chocolate coffee), and foods high in tyramine (organ meats, cured meats, cheese, raisins, avocados, and soy).
   c. Foods high in vitamin K (broccoli, spinach, Brussels sprouts, cauliflower, kale) and vitamin E supplements.
   d. Milk products and vitamins, vitamins and minerals containing iron, and caffeine.

118. A 32-year-old woman with borderline personality disorder and a history of attempted suicide has been married for 8 years, and her husband is filing for divorce. She was found wandering in a state of confused panic about her neighborhood and brought to the ED. She feels extremely anxious and abandoned. Which initial intervention is appropriate for this emotional crisis?
   a. Stay with the patient and reassure her.
   b. Administer anti-anxiety medication.
   c. Provide positive reinforcement.
   d. Draw up a no-suicide contract.

119. The psychiatric/mental health nurse observes that a 50-year-old male with anxiety disorder seems tense and states, "I notice you are wringing your hands." Which therapeutic communication technique does this exemplify?
   a. Presenting reality.
   b. Making observations.
   c. Reflecting.
   d. Giving recognition.

120. A patient refuses to participate in a group activity, stating, "I don't want to do this!" When using the SOAP format, this statement would be documented in:
   a. Subjective.
   b. Objective
   c. Assessment.
   d. Plan.

121. The type of group therapy in which the members share some key features, such as the same diagnosis, but differ in age or gender is:
   a. Homogeneous.
   b. Heterogeneous.
   c. Open.
   d. Mixed.

122. Mike Brown has completed gender reassignment surgery (male-to-female) and is now legally Mikaela Brown. Mikaela states that she is still attracted to females and not males. Her sexual orientation should be most appropriately classified as:
   a. Lesbian.
   b. Heterosexual.
   c. Homosexual.
   d. Bisexual.

123. When instituting suicide precautions, which patient is likely at highest risk?
   a. A 15-year-old girl who overdosed on aspirin and then told her best friend
   b. A 50-year-old woman who overdosed on pills and alcohol while her family was present
   c. A 26-year-old man who threatened to jump out of a second-story window
   d. A 38-year-old man who shot himself in the chest while alone at home

124. When evaluating outcomes data for evidence-based practice, the type of data that includes measures of mortality, longevity, and cost-effectiveness is:
   a. Clinical.
   b. Psychosocial.
   c. Integrative.
   d. Physiological.

125. During the initial patient interview, the patient jumps from one topic to another with little coherence. The term for this type of communication is:
   a. Word salad.
   b. Flight of ideas.
   c. Evasion.
   d. Loose association.

126. When describing extrapyramidal effects of drugs, the following term refers to the inability to start a movement:
   a. Akinesia
   b. Akathisia
   c. Dystonia
   d. Bradykinesia

127. Which of the following provides unit level data regarding psychiatric physical and sexual assaults to help determine the quality of nursing care?
   a. National Center for Health Statistics (NCHS)
   b. National Database of Nursing Quality Indicators (NDNQI)
   c. National Death Index (NDI)
   d. MedlinePlus

128. The purpose of the Life Safety Code® is:
   a. Disease prevention.
   b. Accident prevention.
   c. Infection control.
   d. Fire prevention.

129. When determining the burden of proof for acts of negligence, risk management would classify willfully providing inadequate care while disregarding the safety and security of another as:
   a. Negligent conduct.
   b. Gross negligence.
   c. Contributory negligence.
   d. Comparative negligence.

130. Which of the following diets may decrease excretion of lithium and cause toxic levels to develop?
   a. Low fat
   b. Low protein
   c. Low carbohydrate
   d. Low sodium

131. When the psychiatric/mental health nurse delegates a task to another healthcare provider, the most important consideration when choosing the right person is:
    a. Availability.
    b. Reliability.
    c. Education/Skills.
    d. Years of experience.

132. Two staff nurses in the psychiatric unit disagree about the best way to carry out duties, resulting in ongoing conflict and refusal to work together. The first step in resolving this conflict is to:
    a. Allow both individuals to present their side of the conflict without bias.
    b. Encourage them to reach a compromise.
    c. Tell them they are violating professional standards of conduct.
    d. Make a decision about the matter.

133. Which of the following tests is most accurate for determining acute changes in nutritional status to monitor dietary compliance for a patient with anorexia?
    a. Transferrin
    b. Total protein
    c. Albumin
    d. Prealbumin

134. For recertification, what percentage of continuing education hours must be from formally approved providers?
    a. 25%
    b. 50%
    c. 51%
    d. 75%

135. Suicide attempts during hospitalization have resulted in an average of 7 extra days of hospitalization, with extra cost of approximately $14,000 for each attempt. Various interventions are being considered. The method used to determine monetary savings resulting from planned interventions is:
    a. Cost-benefit analysis.
    b. Cost-effective analysis.
    c. Efficacy study.
    d. Cost-utility analysis.

136. During the initial assessment, a 75-year-old female states she has had one fall in the last 4 months but had no residual injury. What, if any, further testing is immediately indicated?
    a. No further testing
    b. Gait, balance, and get-up-and-go
    c. X-ray of hips and spine
    d. Bone mass density testing

137. The most important criterion for determining the degree of a patient's pain is:
    a. Physical indication, such as grimacing or guarding.
    b. Moaning.
    c. Patient report.
    d. Patient history.

138. A 22-year-old female is receiving haloperidol for schizoaffective disorder. She was admitted to the psychiatric unit with delusional thinking, rapid disorganized speech, irritability, and lethargy. She has begun slapping at her face repeatedly. Which assessment tool is most indicated?
    a. Abnormal Involuntary Movement Scale (AIMS)
    b. CAGE
    c. Mini-mental state exam (MMSE)
    d. Confusion Assessment Method (CAM)

139. A psychiatric/mental health nurse engaged as a consultation liaison is expected to primarily:
    a. Meet with consultants in the psychiatric unit.
    b. Coordinate activities of different consultants.
    c. Serve as a mentor to other nurses in the medical, surgical, and obstetric units.
    d. Assess psychiatric disorders and emotional needs of medical, surgical, and obstetric patients.

140. The psychiatric/mental health nurse is meeting with 10 staff members to review quality improvement data. The most effective initial presentation method is to:
    a. Make copies of raw data and place in bound notebooks to give to staff.
    b. Provide a PowerPoint® presentation that summarizes the data of the report.
    c. Ask staff members what information they'd like to have and proceed from there.
    d. Read a summary of the report to the staff members.

141. Under the NANDA-I Approved Nursing Diagnoses categories, "anxiety" is an example of which type of diagnosis?
    a. Risk
    b. Health promotion
    c. Actual
    d. Syndrome

142. A 45-year-old male with bipolar disorder has been hospitalized for two weeks, and has exhibited signs of methamphetamine abuse and withdrawal but denies taking drugs. The best drug-screening test to evaluate pre-admission use of methamphetamine at this point is:
    a. Urine.
    b. Blood.
    c. Sweat.
    d. Hair.

143. Recommendations for the use of restraint and seclusion in pediatric patients limit the time children ages 9 to 17 should be restrained and/or secluded to no longer than:
a. One hour.
b. Two hours.
c. Four hours.
d. Six hours.

144. An 80-year-old woman has sudden onset of right-sided paresis, short-term memory loss, depression, right visual field defect, and mild expressive aphasia, indicating a possible stroke. The most likely part of the brain affected is the:
a. Right hemisphere.
b. Left hemisphere.
c. Brain stem.
d. Cerebellum.

145. A 62-year-old homeless man hospitalized for schizophrenia is to be discharged but has no place to go and no income. Which of the following is of primary importance in preparing for discharge?
a. Specific directions for medication or treatments, including side effects.
b. Information sheets outlining signs for all risk factors.
c. List of safe shelters and assistance in applying for welfare assistance or Social Security.
d. Follow-up appointment dates, with physicians, labs, or other healthcare providers.

146. A 55-year-old patient with paranoid delusions had an admitting white blood cell (WBC) count with 6,000 WBCs, 4% bands, and 55% neutrophils. A second blood count was done when the patient became increasingly lethargic and refused to eat because "the food is poisoning me." The follow-up blood count showed 15,00 WBCs, 10% bands, and 65% neutrophils. The most likely cause is:
a. Bacterial infection.
b. Viral infection.
c. Dehydration.
d. Allergic reaction.

147. According to the American Academy of Child & Adolescent Psychiatry (AACAP), electroconvulsive therapy (ECT) is indicated for adolescents under the following conditions:
a. Initial treatment for mania with psychotic features.
b. Patient preference.
c. Lack of response to at least 2 drug trials combined with other therapy.
d. Initial treatment of severe psychotic disorders.

148. A 28-year-old patient has a dual diagnosis of bipolar disorder and substance abuse (cocaine, alcohol). The first outcome goal is for the patient to:
a. Interact appropriately with others.
b. Become active in drug- and alcohol-free activities.
c. Develop a plan for activities during free time.
d. Take only medications that have been prescribed.

149. For quality/performance improvement, the best tool to determine methods to streamline processes is:
   a. Root cause analysis.
   b. Tracer methodology.
   c. Family survey.
   d. Staff survey.

150. A 68-year-old male with moderate Alzheimer's disease is usually docile but becomes very agitated and disruptive during mealtimes in the communal dining room. The initial step to handling this is to:
   a. Provide meals in the patient's room.
   b. Encourage more participation by giving patient meal choices.
   c. Request a physician order for antipsychotic medication.
   d. Observe the patient carefully to determine what triggers the agitation.

Answers and Explanations

1. A: According to Title II and Title III of the Americans with Disabilities Act, an emotional comfort animal does not qualify as a service animal. Service animals must actually provide some type of active service and must be canine, although special requests can be made to qualify miniature horses. Psychiatric services dogs, on the other hand, are qualified and may be trained to identify oncoming psychiatric episodes, they may remind the patient to take medications, interrupt self-injurious behavior, or protect disoriented patients from danger.

2. C: If, on physical exam, a patient with chronic alcohol use disorder exhibits ophthalmoplegia, ataxia, and confusion with stupor and somnolence, the most likely cause is vitamin B deficiency, primarily thiamine (vitamin B1). These symptoms are the typical triad associated with Wernicke disease. Patients often also exhibit signs of Korsakoff's psychosis with anterograde and retrograde amnesia and confabulation, so this combination is referred to as Wernicke-Korsakoff syndrome. These conditions are life threatening if not treated aggressively with thiamine replacement.

3. B: If a patient with autism spectrum disorder level 1 cannot judge the intention behind commands, becomes distraught over simple directions ("eat your lunch now"), and ignores important directions ("leave by the fire exit"), the term for this type of deficit is mind blindness. This same deficit interferes with patients' abilities to recognize faces. Mind blindness may contribute to impaired social interaction. A meltdown may begin with a tantrum but is more intense as the patient totally loses control and may endanger self or others. Stereotypy is rigid obsessive behavior. These deficits all result in impaired social interaction.

4. D: For a 35-year-old recently widowed woman with severe anxiety and panic attacks left with few employable skills, little money, and 3 children, the primary need related to Maslow's Hierarchy of Needs is likely safety/security. Although the patient apparently had a stable and happy marriage, meeting the love/belonging need, and while lower needs must be fulfilled before higher needs, it is not uncommon for people to regress under stress. Now, the patient has real concerns about supporting and providing safely for her family, so she must meet the need for safety/security before she can again progress to the next level.

5. A: The evidence-based therapy recommended for adolescents with anorexia nervosa is family-based therapy. Cognitive behavioral therapy is used with adults. Because adolescents with anorexia are not able to make good decisions about food or eating, the family is mobilized to assist the patient and carry out therapeutic interventions, such as refeeding and other efforts to restore weight to a healthy level. Because caloric intake must be high to increase weight, the family must be physically present and must monitor each meal, regardless of the time needed for the adolescent to finish eating.

6. B: If a therapist is basing therapy on the theory of behaviorism, the psychiatric and mental health nurse expects that the focus of the patient's care will be on providing positive reinforcement. Behaviorism is based on the theory that patients are essentially passive and behavior results from stimulus and response. Behaviors that are met with positive reinforcement are likely to be repeated. However, behaviors met with negative reinforcement are also likely to be repeated.

7. C: Secondary prevention requires some type of intervention to deal with inappropriate behavior, such as by working with the patient to modify negative behavior. The adolescent patient may receive secondary prevention measures (treatment) in the community or as an inpatient. If the patient is hospitalized, the psychiatric and mental health nurse focuses on helping the patient learn more appropriate problem- solving skills and helping the patient (and family) stabilize crisis situations.

8. A: A useful exercise for a patient who has perfectionist tendencies and unrealistic expectations of himself and others is to make a list of those things in his life that are in his control (diet, exercise, tasks) and those things that are outside his control (weather, workload, other people). The lists then can serve as a starting point for a discussion because they likely include those things that have been causes for concern to the patient.

9. C: If the psychiatric and mental health nurse believes that the interdisciplinary team is using an unfair approach to assigning workloads to team members, the best response is to ask the team to discuss a different approach. When a conflict arises, it should be dealt with directly rather than simply trying to think differently about the issue, but a negative approach (telling the team that the current approach is unfair or appealing to the department head) may make team members defensive and/or angry and less open to change.

10. D: The values clarification process has three steps: (1) choosing, (2) prizing, and (3) acting:
- Choosing: Considering options and freely choosing a value that feels appropriate for the individual rather than one imposed by others.
- Prizing: Feeling positive about the value and explaining or justifying the value to others.
- Acting: Applying the value to life experiences and interactions with others.

When facilitating the values clarification process with patients, it's important to avoid imposing personal values on the patient.

11. B: If a patient states, "I don't understand. My daughter said that she had to leave town," an appropriate clarifying question would be "Are you confused because you don't know why she had to leave town?" Clarifying questions are utilized to ensure that the listener has understood the meaning (as opposed to just the words) of the patient's statement. Clarifying questions often contain some paraphrase of what the patient has stated and may include such phrases as "Did I understand you to say...?" or "Did you say...?"

12. A: Long-stay inpatients may be referred to a "hospital hostel" program in order to learn living skills such as cooking and cleaning. A hospital hostel program is a separate unit contained within a facility. This unit for long-term patients with severe mental health problems is designed to be less institutional and more like a group home experience. Patients are assisted to develop skills that allow them to improve functioning and, in some cases, transition to community housing.

13. C: One of the primary purposes of partial hospitalization is to monitor the effectiveness of drugs. Partial hospitalization programs provide treatment during the day or evening and are used as a transitional placement for a patient integrating into the community. Administering and monitoring of medications is often done in partial hospitalization

programs. The programs may vary widely in the other services offered, but many programs offer group and individual therapy as well as social skills training and daily living skills training.

14. C: One of the characteristics of an evolving consumer household is that the patient doesn't have to move from home to another. The evolving consumer household is a permanent group home that allows the patient to transition from dependence to increasing levels of independence within the same environment rather than having to move as the person transitions from one level of care to another. Adjusting to new living situations is often stressful for a patient who must adapt to multiple changes at the same time.

15. D: According to Piaget, adulthood begins when the person is able to reason systematically about abstract concepts. Piaget's 4 stages of cognitive development include sensorimotor (birth to 2 years), preoperational (2 to 6 years), concrete operational (6 to 11 years), and formal operational (11 through adulthood). Piaget believed that childhood ended with movement to the formal operational stage although Piaget recognized that not everyone completes the tasks at each stage of development and, thus, not everyone cognitively moves into adulthood.

16. A: A characteristic of an open group is that meetings continue indefinitely. In an open group, membership may vary widely as new patients are free to enter the group, drop out, or move on. A closed group, on the other hand, usually involves the same members, who must approve new members, and meets for a specified number of sessions, such as an 8-week course on managing symptoms for a group of patients with bipolar disorder.

17. B: The purpose of a Snoezelen room is to reduce anxiety and improve communication and functioning. Snoezelen rooms are controlled multisensory environments (MSE). The rooms contain multiple different types of lighting, sounds, music, smells, and textures that can all be manipulated to provide an individualized experience for the patient. The environment should be essentially neutral (neither positive nor negative) and focused on the patient and the patient's preferences. Snoezelen rooms are often used with patients on the autism spectrum and those with dementia or traumatic brain injuries.

18. A: If a psychiatric and mental health nurse working with a 28-year-old female patient with bulimia nervosa finds a container of laxatives hidden in the patient's bed linens, the best response is to tell the patient directly about finding the laxatives without making a judgmental statement. If consequences for violating rules have been established, then those consequences should be applied. Establishing an honest relationship is essential to the development of trust between the patient and the nurse.

19. D: If a patient has received long-term treatment with haloperidol as an antipsychotic agent and has developed repetitive behaviors, including tongue thrusting, lip smacking, and hair pulling, the most likely cause is tardive dyskinesia (TD), which is related to use of conventional antipsychotics. TD may result in permanent non-voluntary movements. Symptoms are often irreversible but stopping or changing the medication may reduce symptoms. Patients must be monitored carefully for initial indications of TD so that medications can be changed before symptoms become severe.

20. C: Because experiential readiness to learn relates to the experiences the patient has had, the factor that is most likely to negatively impact a patient's experiential readiness to learn

is if the patient flunked out of high school. This experience may lead the patient to believe that he/she is incapable of learning. An IQ of 68 may impact the patient's knowledge readiness because the patient may lack the ability to learn complex material. Anxiety about learning may impact the patient's emotional readiness to learn.

21. B: If a patient is to receive an SSRI for depression that has been associated with long QT syndrome (LQTS) and tachycardia characterized by *torsade de pointes*, the patient should have a baseline ECG to evaluate for congenital LQTS, periodic ECGs after therapy is initiated, and a careful personal and family history completed, with special attention to cardiac abnormalities. LQTS may be induced by dozens of drugs, including SSRIs and antipsychotic medications, especially in patients with preexisting congenital abnormalities.

22. D: If a patient has been prescribed chlorpromazine hydrochloride, an antipsychotic, the nurse should advise the patient to avoid sun exposure, as photosensitivity reactions of the skin may occur. When outside or exposed to sun, patients should wear sun block and protective clothing. Chlorpromazine is more likely to cause photosensitivity than other medications in the same class. Patients should also avoid alcohol while taking the drug and should avoid activities that require good coordination, especially in the initial weeks of therapy.

23. A: With rational emotive behavior therapy (REBT), the model suggests that (A) adversity (activating event) and (C) consequences are strongly influenced by (B) beliefs about the event. According to this model of therapy, people innately have both rational and irrational tendencies, so if the person has irrational beliefs about an activating event, then the consequences result in feelings of defeat, while if he person has rational beliefs, the consequences are more likely to be seen as constructive.

24. C: Considering the therapeutic nurse-patient relationship as described by Peplau, when the psychiatric and mental health nurse encourages the patient to express feelings about an event, the role the nurse is serving in is the role of counselor, which includes other experiences that promote health. Other roles include stranger (offering general acceptance and courtesy), resource person (providing answers to questions), teacher (helping the patient to learn), leader (providing direction), and surrogate (assuming the role of another, parent, sibling, patient).

25. B: The best response to a patient experiencing auditory hallucinations, saying "Don't you hear them?" is to state "I know the voices seem real to you, but I don't hear them." This response validates the patient's perception and real fear of the voices ("I know the voices seem real to you") while orienting the patient to reality ("I don't hear them"). The psychiatric and mental health nurse should speak in a calm voice and avoid standing too close to or touching the patient without permission, as these actions may increase the patient's fear and anxiety.

26. A: The statement by a patient that is most likely to indicate suicidal ideation and risk for suicide is "My children would be better off without me." When a patient makes a statement indicating possible suicidal ideation, the psychiatric and mental health nurse should address it immediately by asking if the patient has thoughts about dying and if the patient has a plan. Patients who have formulated a plan (such as taking an overdose of medications) are at higher risk than those who simply think about wanting to die.

27. D: With a patient with schizophrenia and a nursing diagnosis of impaired verbal communication, a technique used to show empathy and encourage communication is verbalizing the implied, which is stating verbally what the patient's words or actions imply. This technique may be used for patients who are completely mute. For example, if a patient is cowering and avoiding eye contact, the nurse may say, "Are you feeling frightened?" or "I can see that you are frightened."

28. C: Delusion of reference: Patient believes everything in the environment references her, such as the patient believing that messages are being sent to her in newspapers, magazines, radio, and television and that she must decipher them. Delusion of persecution: Patient believes others intend to harm her. Delusion of control: Patient believes other people or objects control her actions. Delusion of grandeur: Patient believes she is an important person or being, such as God.

29. B: Perseveration: Patient repeats the same word phrase over and over, such as "cake," in response to a question. Associative looseness: Patient shifts comments from one topic to another but is unaware the ideas may be incoherent. Tangentiality: Patient introduces unrelated topics and never returns to the point of the communication. Echolalia: Patient repeats words or phrases that the patient hears. For example, if a psychiatric and mental health nurse states, "It's time to go to bed, "the patient might repeat "it's time to go to bed" over and over or may shorten it to "bed, bed, bed, bed."

30. A: Auditory hallucinations: Patient hears voices or other sounds, such as music or clicks. This is the most common type of hallucination experienced by psychiatric patients. Visual hallucinations: Patient sees formed or unformed images, such as people, animals, and flashes of light. Tactile hallucinations: Patient has false perception of touch, such as the feeling that something is crawling under the patient's skin. Olfactory hallucination: Patient has false perception of smells. Gustatory: Patient has false perception of taste.

31. D: Emotional ambivalence: Patient has opposite emotions about the same thing and cannot, therefore, make even a simple decision, such as choosing between an egg and toast or cereal for breakfast. Depersonalization: Patient experiences feelings of unreality, such as seeing the self from a distance or perceiving distortion in the body. Anhedonia: Patient is unable to experience pleasure. Regression: Patient retreats to an earlier stage of development as a coping mechanism.

32. C: Disturbed thought processes: Patient cannot trust and may experience panic with behavior that may include delusional thinking, decreased volition, impaired problem solving, impaired abstract thinking, and suspicion of others. Disturbed sensory perception: Patient perceives incoming stimuli abnormally and exhibits distorted response. Social isolation: Patient has impaired or absent ability to interact with others. Self-care deficit: Patient has impaired or absent ability to carry out self-care activities, such as bathing.

33. A: Illusion: Patient misinterprets real external stimuli, such as perceiving the picture of the red roses as a monster with blood dripping from its mouth. Delusion: Patient has false personal beliefs despite evidence to the contrary, such as a somatic delusion in which the patient has false ideas about the functioning of his/her body. Hallucination: Patient experiences false sensory perceptions (auditory, visual, tactile, gustatory, and olfactory). Magical thinking: Patient believes that thoughts have power to control others, situations, or things.

34. D: Sublimation: The patient redirects socially unacceptable impulses to acceptable actions, such as when the victim of a crime redirects anger toward becoming an advocate for other victims. Regression: The patient retreats to an earlier stage of development, such as by being more dependent. Suppression: The patient voluntarily blocks unpleasant emotions, such as by refusing to think about an event. Repression: The patient involuntarily blocks unpleasant emotions, such as being unable to remember being raped.

35. B: Intellectualism: Using rational intellectual processes to deal with stress and loss, such as by discussing positive aspects of being single. Displacement: Transferring feelings from one person or thing to another, such as being angry with a boss and taking the anger out on a spouse. Denial: Completely refusing to acknowledge a situation that is stressful, such as ignoring a child's drug use. Rationalization: Attempting to find excuses for unacceptable behavior or feelings, such as drinking to relieve the stress of work.

36. A: If the psychiatric and mental health nurse is teaching an unmotivated patient about managing her disorder and medications, the best approach is probably to provide short lessons and assignments because lack of motivation often corresponds to short attention span. Illustrated materials may not always be appropriate, and the nurse should avoid punishing the patient, as this may further decrease her motivation to learn. Independent study materials require motivation to start with or the patient won't do the work needed.

37. C: The statement by the psychiatric and mental health nurse that indicates that the nurse is fulfilling the role of resource person is: "Let me show you around and answer any questions you might have." The roles of resource person and teacher sometimes overlap to a degree. As a resource person, the nurse should be available to orient the patient to the environment and situation and to apprise the patient of the resources (including services) that are available. In responding to questions, the nurse may assume the role of teacher when providing information the patient should retain.

38. B: During the stage of toddlerhood, the child should learn to delay gratification and feel satisfied when delaying self-gratification is pleasing to others. If patients have not completed tasks of toddlerhood, as adults they may use exploitive and manipulative behavior with others, exhibit envy and suspiciousness toward others, hoard, exhibit miserliness, exhibit inordinate neatness/punctuality, have difficulty relating to others, and alter personality characteristics to fit the situation. A patient who has not completed toddlerhood tasks requires complete acceptance in order to feel safe and secure.

39. D: Characteristics of crises include:
- Crises are personal in nature. What one person considers a crisis may be only an annoyance to another person or of no concern at all.
- Precipitating events are always identifiable.
- Crises are always acute and not chronic and are usually resolved in a fairly short duration of time.
- All people experience some type of crisis at one time in their lives or another although not all crises are associated with psychopathology.
- A crisis may provide the potential for psychological growth or impairment, depending on the individual response.

40. C: When creating an environment conducive to learning for one-on-one instruction for a patient with anxiety disorder (or any other individual patient), the best environment is the patient's preference. While patients with anxiety often prefer a quiet secluded area, some may find background music soothing while others may find it distracting. Some may feel more secure with bright lighting and others with dim lighting. Adolescents and young adults, for example, are often used to studying with loud music in the background and don't find that distracting while many others do.

41. A: The type of exercise that may reduce symptoms of anxiety and depression is aerobic exercise, such as jogging, walking, gardening, and riding bicycles. Psychiatric and mental health patients often lead relatively sedentary lives because of their symptoms and adverse effects associated with their medications, increasing their risks for obesity, diabetes, and heart disease. An exercise regimen should be part of lifestyle changes and should include a minimum of 30 minutes of aerobic exercise at least 3 times weekly.

42. D: Allowing another nurse not assigned to the patient to read the patient's records is a violation of HIPAA regulations because it violates confidentiality. Only staff members with a need to access the patient's records (such as the psychiatrist, therapist, and assigned nursing personnel) may legally access a patient's records. HIPAA requires that access to electronic health records be with a unique identifier and password, which should not be shared with others. Additionally, the computer screen should not be visible to unauthorized people.

43. B: If a patient is able to read printed directions out loud with minimal difficulty, this means that the patient is able to decode words. To test for comprehension, after the patient completes the reading, the psychiatric and mental health nurse should ask the patient to paraphrase the directions to determine if the patient was able to understand what was read. Delaying the quiz for 2 days tests retention rather than comprehension. Some people may comprehend well but have poor retention because of impaired memory.

44. D: Most people with reasonable cognitive ability understand that smoking is bad for their health, so threatening them or scaring them is not likely to motivate them to quit. Realistically, success rates for smoking cessation are often low, so the psychiatric and mental health nurse should consider that not everyone will be successful at quitting and should provide information as a preventive measure about symptoms of concern, such as increasing cough, purulent or bloody sputum, and increased shortness of breath.

45. C: Because this patient was admitted on a 72-hour hold instead of voluntarily, the patient may have little motivation to change behavior. The priority resource is the methadone program as this program may allow the patient to stop heroin use. Narcotics Anonymous® is a good self-help group, but the patient should be motivated to attend, although sometimes attendance is required by the court. Group therapy is also a good resource, but the patient probably needs to be off of drugs before she is willing to attend. Home health agencies may not provide the services needed.

46. B: While most screening for intimate partner abuse focuses on females age 18 or older, all female patients ages 14 and older should be screened, as many very young females engage in sexual relationships, and this makes them vulnerable to intimate partner abuse. Additionally, some screening may also be appropriate for males, who are sometimes also

the victims of abuse. Intimate partner abuse also occurs in same sex relationships, both male and female, so healthcare providers should be alert to those possibilities.

47. D: The behavior that would differentiate aggression from anger is making verbal threats, as this often means that the patient's anger is escalating, and the person's response may be disproportionate to the situation. Other indications of aggression include restless behavior and pacing back and forth, shouting in a loud voice, and using obscenities. The person may be very suspicious and exhibit disturbed thought processes and increased agitation and overreaction to stimuli. Aggressive individuals almost always have intent to hurt someone or something.

48. C: The best tool to ensure medication adherence is patient education. Patients should understand why the medication is prescribed, the dosage, and the schedule of administration. Additionally, the patient should know what to do if a dosage is missed and what steps to take to refill the prescription. The patient should understand the adverse effects that can occur with the drug and any possible interactions with other substances, including food and other drugs. The patient should have a schedule for any monitoring that is necessary, such as drug levels or white blood cell counts.

49. A: Under provisions of the Americans with Disabilities Act (ADA) related to people with psychiatric disabilities, employers are required to provide reasonable accommodations. This does not mean the ADA requires hiring people with psychiatric disabilities, holding a position open, or providing any and all requests that people make. The employee must still be able to carry out the job for which the person was hired, although accommodations such as flexible work hours or break time and a more quiet space to work, are reasonable.

50. D: A realistic goal of relapse prevention therapy (RPT) is to help patients deal with the potential for relapse. RPT is sometimes used as the primary substance abuse treatment but may also be used for aftercare to encourage compliance. The program uses cognitive (reframing) and behavioral (meditation, exercise) techniques to teach patients to understand the process of relapse, identify situations that place them at risk of relapse, cope with cravings, recover after relapse and continue the program, and learn to lead a more satisfying and balanced life.

51. B: In order for a patient with a terminal disease to be admitted to a hospice program under Medicare, the physician must certify that the patient's death is expected within 6 months. However, since the time of death is not always predictable, the patient can be certified for two 90-day periods initially followed by an unlimited number of 60-day periods, although at the beginning of each 60-day period, the physician must again certify that the patient's death is expected within 6 months.

52. A: If a patient who has been using heroin is admitted to the psychiatric unit, the patient is likely to exhibit withdrawal symptoms within 6 to 12 hours after the last dose of heroin because heroin is relatively short acting. Withdrawal symptoms usually peak within 1 to 3 days and subside by the end of a week. Typical withdrawal symptoms include nausea and vomiting, abdominal cramping, myopathy, dysphoric mood, fever, diarrhea, rhinorrhea, and insomnia.

53. C: The primary reason that milieu therapy (therapeutic community) is less frequently used as a therapeutic approach currently is that the length of stay in psychiatric units has

decreased with the emphasis on medical treatment and short stay. Milieu therapy requires that all aspects of a patient's environment serve to help socialize and treat the patient, but the patient usually only begins to benefit from the socialization aspects of milieu therapy after being stabilized, at which point the patient is generally discharged and treated as an outpatient.

54. D: If a patient has difficulty with both verbal and nonverbal communication that is appropriate for the social context, is unable to match communication to the needs of the listener, and has difficulty recognizing clues for turn-taking but exhibits no additional behavior associated with autism spectrum disorder, these symptoms are characteristic of social (pragmatic) communication disorder. Autism spectrum disorder is characterized by more intense verbal and nonverbal communication problems as well as repetitive motor movements, fixated interests, and abnormal response to sensory input, with the level depending on the degree of severity.

55. A: The primary components of dialectical behavioral therapy (DBT) used to treat borderline personality disorder are:
- Psychotherapy: This type of CBT focuses on adaptive behaviors by exploring events and discussing alternative responses to help the patient cope with personal perception of trauma. Problems are focused on in a priority order, beginning with suicidal behavior and therapy-interfering behavior before quality of life issues, post-traumatic stress, self respect, acquisition of behavior skills, and patient-centered goals
- Group therapy: Focuses on behavioral skills, including distractions and self-soothing techniques as well as accepting reality.

56. D: If a patient with antisocial personality disorder tells the psychiatric and mental health nurse (who is sensitive about her weight) that other staff members are making fun of her appearance and state that she is "fat and lazy," the nurse should remain calm, avoid showing a reaction, and advise the patient that his comments are inappropriate. Pathological personality traits common to antisocial personality disorder include antagonism characterized by manipulation, deceit, callousness, and hostility. The patient often uses dishonesty, lack of feelings, and hostility to manipulate others.

57. B: If a patient was diagnosed with major depressive disorder after 6 months of depression but did not respond to a trial of an SSRI or another trial of an SNRI, the most likely next step is to explore the possible diagnosis of bipolar disorder because the depressive episodes associated with bipolar disorder do not necessarily respond to antidepressants. Interviews with family members may provide a family history of bipolar disorder or evidence of mania or hypomania that the patient may have not recognized. Early onset (adolescence to young adulthood) is also characteristic of bipolar disorder.

58. C: The dissociative subtype of post-traumatic stress disorder (PTSD), a new classification of PTSD in the *DSM-5*, is characterized by:
- Depersonalization: This is an out-of-the-body experience in which the patient feels outside of the physical body, decreasing the physical and emotional response normally associated with stress.
- Derealization: The patient feels as though in a dream state and as though the events surrounding the patient are not real, resulting in a muted emotional response.

59. B: The statement by a patient in CBT for major depressive disorder suggesting that the patient is applying principles learned in therapy is, "I can't fix this situation, so I'm going to think about taking a vacation." One of the goals of CBT is to help patients to think differently about situations and to use thought-stopping exercises when they begin to obsess over problems, such as a situation they can't fix. Patients use imagery, such as imagining taking a vacation, to help to have more positive thoughts.

60. A: Interpersonal therapy is generally most effective for depressive episodes associated with specific situations (such as grief) and is usually of short duration (six 20-minute sessions). During therapy, the focus is on one issue, such as conflicts, changing roles, or grief. The patient is helped to develop specific goals, and the therapist confronts the patient when the patient's behavior does not facilitate reaching these goals. Patients are encouraged to remain focused on the problem and associated concrete feelings rather than abstract feelings.

61. C: An example of self-harm is when a patient cuts herself on the legs with a razor. Suicidal attempts are not classified as self-harm because the intent is different. Self-harm always involves some type of physical violence directed at the self and is carried out by the person intentionally. Negative thoughts, such as a patient telling herself she is a failure, are not classified as self-harm. Body piercing, tattooing, and other behaviors that alter the body are not considered self-harm although they may, at times, be harmful.

62. D: According to Erikson's stages of human development, the key event for people between the ages of 40 to 65 years (generativity vs. stagnation), which is classified as middle adulthood, is parenting, as people of this age are increasingly interested in providing guidance for the next generation. People are generally productive in their work life and may be more involved in community affairs than previously. If people feel unproductive during this stage of development, this leads to stagnation.

63. D: If a psychiatric and mental health nurse is physically attacked by a patient and the nurse suffers a broken arm as a result, this would be a Serious Reportable Event (SRE) in the category of *potential criminal event*. It is "potential" because it may not be criminal if the patient were delusional, for example. Other potentially criminal events include care ordered or provided by someone impersonating a healthcare worker, abduction of a patient or resident, and sexual assault of a patient or staff member.

64. A: The lithium level for maintenance should be 0.5 to 1.5 mEq/L. If the level increases to 1.5 to 2 mEq/L, then the next dose of medication should be withheld and the serum level of the drug tested. A further increase to 2 to 3 mEq/L is of considerable concern as the patient may exhibit moderate signs of toxicity. The patient requires immediate IV fluids as well as withholding of lithium. A level of 3 mEq/L or above is life threatening and requires emergent intervention, sometimes including dialysis to lower lithium levels.

65. C: A common myth associated with suicide is that people who commit suicide always do so to hurt only themselves. While sometimes true, in fact, some people go to great lengths to ensure that their suicides will be hurtful to others, such as when a person waits to shoot himself until a family member is present to observe or when a person leaves a note blaming someone else for the suicide. Other myths are that people who talk about suicide don't attempt it, and once a risk of suicide, always a risk.

66. B: If a patient expresses lack of control over her life and personal situation and doesn't participate in her own care or decision-making, an appropriate nursing diagnosis is powerlessness. Interventions include encouraging the patient to verbalize feelings, acknowledging the patient's personal knowledge of her situation, promoting the patient's sense of autonomy, and encouraging the patient to identify her own strengths. An expected outcome is that the patient will begin to identify ways of achieving control and to participate in decision-making.

67. B: If, while conducting a peer review, the psychiatric and mental health nurse observes the other nurse using non-therapeutic communication techniques with a patient, the best response is to discuss the observations at a post-review meeting. The other nurse is not being negligent, so there is no need to intervene immediately or report the observation. During the discussion, the psychiatric and mental health nurse should prompt the other nurse by stating, "How did you feel about your communication with the patient?"

68. C: If a patient has an intellectual disability and an IQ of 45 (moderate disability), a realistic maximal expectation is that the patient may be capable of working in a sheltered workshop, as the patient should be capable of performing some activities independently while requiring some supervision. The patient should be able to achieve an academic level comparable to second grade. The patient may exhibit some speech impediments and have difficulty with peer relationships because of inability to understand or adhere to social conventions.

69. D: According to the American Nurses Association *Code of Ethics,* the responsible agent for the psychiatric and mental health nurse's nursing practice when the nurse is employed in a hospital is the individual nurse. The nurse also remains responsible for tasks carried out by someone to whom the nurse has delegated the task. The primary commitment of the nurse should always be to the patient, and the nurse must serve as an advocate for the rights, safety, and health of the patient.

70. A: If a patient's family caregivers are interesting in taking classes or training to better help them assist the patient and cope more effectively with the patient's illness, the most appropriate referral is to the National Alliance on Mental Illness (NAMI). NAMI's Family-to-Family program is especially intended for family caregivers of those with severe mental illness. Family-to-Family comprises a 12-week course that is free. NAMI Basics is a course intended for parents/caregivers of children and adolescents with mental illness.

71. C: If a psychiatric and mental health nurse has agreed to formally mentor a newly-graduated registered nurse for a 2-year period, the mentor should plan to meet with the mentee during the first year at least weekly. According to the National Center for Educational Statistics, almost 90% of mentees who met weekly with their mentor felt they had benefited considerably from mentoring while less than 40% felt they had benefited if they met only less frequently.

72. A: A symmetrical pattern of bruising and petechiae up and down the back, chest, and shoulders, and across the forehead probably indicates coining *(Cao gio).* This is a practice that is common in Southeast Asia and can appear as severe bruising, but the bruises are not random in the same way that is expected with abuse. An ointment is first applied to the skin, which is then rubbed firmly with a coin (or sometimes a spoon) until discoloration occurs as a method to rid the body of "bad blood" that may be causing illness.

73. C: A warning sign that a psychiatric and mental health nurse may have breached professional patient-nurse boundaries is when the nurse confides personal or secret information to a patient, such as that the nurse is having financial problems. Acknowledging a personal preference for some types of patients is not a problem unless the nurse shows preference. Spending extra time with a patient in crisis does not breach boundaries, although spending extra time with a patient because of enjoying the patient's company may. Thinking about a patient outside of work may be a breach, although problem-solving thoughts generally are not.

74. D: When a psychiatric and mental health nurse says to a patient, "Tell me about how you were sexually abused by your father," this is an example of the non-therapeutic communication technique of probing. Probing usually involves pushing the patient to answer questions or give details about information the patient would prefer not to divulge or is not yet ready to divulge. Patients may react defensively and feel that the nurse values the patient only for the information and doesn't care about the patient's feelings.

75. C: An example of feedback that is directed at an action that the patient cannot modify is "You have memory problems because of your alcohol abuse" because the patient cannot undo the physical damage that has been caused by any specific action. The patient can modify behavior based on the other feedback. The patient can modify behavior if the patient has made an inappropriate comment, can control or explore the reasons for anger, and can also attempt to make eye contact with the son during a subsequent visit.

76. A: The emphasis of reality therapy (Glasser) is on the present, the here and now, and personal responsibility. Patients examine the ways in which their behavior has interfered with their ability to achieve goals. The view of reality therapy is that the individual is responsible for his or her choice of actions. According to this theory, people are born with 5 basic needs--power, belonging, freedom, fun, and survival—and people develop personality in trying to fulfill these needs. Present behavior is addressed, not past, unless behavior in the past has specifically affected present behavior.

77. A: Considering assertiveness training, an example of "clouding/fogging" in response to the statement, "You should be fired for the way you handled that situation," is "You're right. I could have handled that situation better." Clouding/fogging addresses only part of the issue (handling the situation better) and "clouds" or by-steps the other (should be fired) as a way to assert control of the issue. Other types of assertive responses include agreeing assertively, inquiring assertively, defusing, and responding with irony.

78. D: According to cognitive behavioral therapy (CBT), the type of automatic thought exemplified when a patient states, "My mother thinks I'm a failure," is *mind reading* because the patient is assuming to know what is in another person's mind (although this would not hold true if the mother actually stated that the patient was a failure). An example of discounting positives is, "Of course I passed the test. The teacher made it too easy." All-or-nothing leaves no room for another interpretation: "Everyone knows I'm stupid." Personalizing brings everything back to the individual, "He's successful because of my advice and help."

79. B: The most appropriate tool to differentiate delirium from other types of confusion is the Confusion Assessment Method, which can be used for those without psychiatric training.

The tool covers 9 different factors associated with abnormal behavior: onset, attention, thinking, level of consciousness, orientation, memory, perceptual disturbances, psychomotor abnormalities, and sleep-wake cycle. An acute onset of confusion with fluctuation in attention level and disorganized thoughts or an altered state of consciousness is characteristic of delirium.

80. C: If a patient with substance abuse disorder states he has been using "beanies," the psychiatric and mental health nurse should understand that the patient is referring to methamphetamine, which is also sometimes referred to as "blue devils," "crank," and "crystal" as well as any number of local names. Marijuana is commonly called "weed," "Aunt Mary," "Mary Jane," and "pot." Cocaine may be called many names, including "coke," "blow,", "snow," and "sugar." Heroin may be called "horse," "H," "Aunt Hazel," "smack," and "charley" as well as many less commonly-used names.

81. B: The task that the psychiatric and mental health nurse can delegate to unlicensed assistive personnel (UAP) is taking routine vital signs. Generally, UAP can assist patients with activities of daily living, including personal hygiene, dressing, and ambulating. UAP can transfer patients, assist with meals, help with socialization activities and can reinforce health teaching but cannot be responsible for planning the health teaching. UAP cannot carry out physical or psychosocial assessments and can never give medications to a patient.

82. B: A patient who has been very upset because his girlfriend broke up with him when he was hospitalized is exhibiting *transference* when he begins to follow the psychiatric and mental health nurse, insulting her and suggesting that she is trying to undermine his therapy. Transference is the transfer of feelings (affection or hostility) from one person to another because of unconscious identification. Countertransference is an emotional reaction of the nurse or therapist to the patient.

83. A: In a group process, the three major types of roles that group members assume within the group are:
- Completing group tasks: Roles may include coordinating, evaluating, energizing, orienting, and elaborating:
- Supporting the group process: Roles may include compromising, encouraging, following, harmonizing, and gate keeping.
- Fulfilling personal needs: Roles may include being aggressive, dominating, blocking, help-seeking, monopolizing, seeking recognition, and seducing.

While completing group tasks and supporting group processes function to make the group effective, roles involved in fulfilling personal needs may interfere with the overall functioning of the group.

84. D: The most appropriate intervention for severe confusion and agitation in a patient with a neurocognitive disorder due to Alzheimer's disease is non-pharmacological measures, such as altering the environment, using distraction, allowing the patient to pace, and identifying triggers. Numerous studies have shown that antipsychotics are no better than placebos and result in increased risk and adverse effects. Anticonvulsants also show no benefit. SSRIs have not been shown to reduce agitation, confusion, or depression in patients with Alzheimer's disease.

85. B: Characteristics of binge-eating disorder (BED), which is regular episodes of overeating, include:

- Eating alone out of embarrassment at the amount of food eaten.
- Eating large amounts of food despite no feeling of hunger.
- Eating large amounts of food despite feeling uncomfortably full.
- Eating very rapidly.
- Having feelings of self-disgust and guilt over eating habits.

BED is newly included in the *DSM-5* as a distinct disorder and is considered the most common eating disorder in the United States.

86. C: If a patient has a diagnosis of social isolation, the description that is appropriate to document in the patient's electronic health record (EHR) is, "Patient stays alone in room, stating 'Go away,' when asked to participate in group activities." In documenting, it is important to describe rather than label because labels, such as "withdrawn," "isolating," and "uncooperative" may be interpreted in various ways and do not provide a clear picture of the patient's behavior.

87. D: The four essential components of informed consent before a patient can make a decision about care are:

- Voluntarism: The patient must be free to make the decision without coercion, manipulation, or threats although persuasion may be utilized.
- Competence: The patient must be mentally competent enough to make decisions.
- Disclosure: The healthcare provider must provide full disclosure about treatment, including what comprises the treatment, any alternate options, and the purpose.
- Comprehension: The patient must be able to understand the implications of treatment.

88. A: The organization/agency that provides the Evidence-Based Practices (EBP) Web Guide for treatment of mental and substance abuse disorders is the Substance Abuse and Mental Health Services Administration (SAMHSA). The EBP Web Guide links to other sites that provide evidence-based guidelines that meet criteria for inclusion. Criteria include providing adequate information, containing multiple EBPs, maintaining functional links, providing documents in forms other than just PDF files, and providing the information free of charge. The information is organized by categories: Behavioral Health Area and Intended Age Group.

89. B: If a patient with a substance abuse disorder has a nursing diagnosis of *ineffective coping* in the nursing care plan, an appropriate expected outcome would be "Patient begins to recognize maladaptive behaviors." Other expected outcomes may include participating in treatment programs, abstaining from use of alcohol or drugs, and demonstrating positive coping efforts. Related factors often include increased vulnerability and inadequate support resources. Patients with ineffective coping are often unable to meet obligations of social role and may have difficulty with problem solving and may exhibit destructive behavior to self and others.

90. C: According to Maslow's Hierarchy of Needs, the nursing diagnoses would be prioritized in the following manner (first to last):

- Physiological needs: Sleep deprivation.
- Safety and security needs: Risk for injury.
- Love and belonging: Social isolation.
- Esteem (self and from others): Ineffective coping.

The last need is for self-actualization, but Maslow's Hierarchy of Needs is predicated on the idea that one must meet the needs at one level before progressing to the next level; so many people are never able to meet the needs associated with self-actualization.

91. B: According to the four phases of alcoholic drinking behavior (Jellinek), blackouts are a characteristic of Phase II, Early Alcoholic. Phases:

- Phase I, Pre-alcoholic: Using alcohol to relieve stress (often learned behavior from childhood).
- Phase II, Early Alcoholic: Sneaking drinks, experiencing blackouts, and reacting defensively about drinking.
- Phase III, Crucial: Binge drinking, losing control to physiological dependence, displaying anger and aggression, and showing a willingness to sacrifice almost everything for alcohol.
- Phase IV, Chronic: Disintegrating physically and emotionally, being intoxicated most of the time, and experiencing life-threatening adverse effects.

92. B: Typical behavior associated with intoxication from inhalant use includes belligerence, assaultiveness, impaired judgment, and slurred speech. The person may exhibit impaired gait, tremors, and blurred vision. Users may also experience irritation of the mouth and throat. The symptoms may progress to CNS depression and cardiac dysrhythmias, which can result in death. Intoxication occurs within 5 minutes of use and symptoms persist for 60 to 90 minutes. Inhalants are a popular choice for adolescents because of accessibility.

93. D: Negative symptoms associated with schizophrenia include blunt or flat affect, lack of energy and passivity (anergia), lack of motivation and inability to initiate tasks (avolition), poverty of speech content and speech production, and sudden interruption in speech and thought patterns so that the patient may stop speaking in the middle of an idea when the patient loses track of what he or she was saying (thought stopping). Negative symptoms impair social functioning and the ability to hold a job because of the patient's difficulty with decision-making and communication.

94. C: With obsessive-compulsive disorder (OCD), a common compulsion is repeatedly checking to make sure that the door is locked. Obsessions occur within the mind, such as experiencing unwanted thoughts and being fearful, while compulsions involve the need to carry out an action, such as washing the hands repeatedly, arranging objects in a specific manner, making lists, and tapping. Hoarding may occur with OCD as a compulsion, but it is now considered a separate disorder.

95. B: If a patient has sat in the same chair with the right arm extended for an hour after the phlebotomist extended the arm for a blood draw, this is an example of waxy flexibility, a psychomotor behavior associated with schizophrenia with catatonia. With waxy flexibility, the patient maintains a position initiated by someone else (such as the phlebotomist). This

differs from posturing in that, with posturing, the patient voluntarily assumes abnormal or bizarre postures.

96. A: Because of constant need, homeless people are most likely to be motivated by self-interest, so offering free food, water, and hygiene products is probably the best method to use to encourage participation. While funding may be limited, sometimes community members or organizations such as the Salvation Army® will contribute, so the psychiatric and mental health nurse may need to consider partnering with or working with other community resources, including homeless shelters and food kitchens, as these organizations can refer the homeless.

97. B: Membership in the American Psychiatric Nurses Association (APNA) is available to all licensed registered nurses, regardless of the type of education: RN, BSN, MSN, and DON. Affiliate membership is available to all other mental health professionals (non-nursing), such as occupational therapists. Student memberships are available for students enrolled full-time in a nursing degree program. Retired membership is also available tor nurses who have retired but remain interested in mental health issues. International membership for nurses who reside outside of the United States is also available.

98. C: The most commonly cited barrier to psychiatric treatment for mental health patients at all levels of severity is low perceived need. Patients often believe that they can cope by themselves or that their symptoms are not so severe as to require medical attention. Other barriers include stigma against mental illness although as the public becomes better informed, this is less of a concern than in previous decades. Financial costs and access (lack of transportation or programs) are also factors.

99. D: If a patient who was voluntarily committed to a psychiatric facility wants to leave and is restrained from doing so by a psychiatric and mental health nurse, this may constitute false imprisonment as the patient has the legal right to leave, even against medical advice. Assault and battery may occur if a patient was treated without consent or threatened. Intentional torts are voluntary purposeful actions intended to bring about a physical or mental consequence. Negligence is providing substandard care.

100. A: The electrolyte imbalance of most concern with polydipsia, which is characterized by excessively drinking water >3L per day, is hyponatremia because of the diluting effect that the water has on the blood and the inability of the kidneys to excrete urine fast enough. Polydipsia may occur with schizophrenia as well as in those with developmental disabilities. If untreated, the patient may develop seizures and experience cardiac arrest. Treatment of polydipsia generally requires hospitalization. Clozapine is often used to control symptoms.

101. D: Havighurst's middle age tasks include achieving civic/social responsibility, maintaining an economic standard of living, raising teenagers and teaching them to be responsible adults, developing leisure activity, accepting physiological changes related to aging, and adjusting to aging of parents. Early adulthood tasks include finding a mate, marrying, having and children, managing a home, getting started in an occupation/profession, assuming civic responsibility, and finding a congenial social group. Older adulthood tasks include adjusting to a decrease in physical strength and health, death of a spouse, and life in retirement and reduced income, as well as establishing ties with those in the same age group, meeting social and civic obligations, and establishing satisfactory physical living arrangements.

102. B: Craving for cocaine during withdrawal may be alleviated by bromocriptine (dopamine agonist) 1.5 mg TID. Withdrawal symptoms include cravings, marked depression, suicidal ideation, insomnia, and hyperphagia, so clients must be monitored carefully. Lorazepam is used to control seizures caused by amphetamine use. Antidotes for common drugs and toxins include:

- Opiates: Naloxone (Narcan®).
- Toxic alcohols: Ethanol infusion and/or dialysis.
- Acetaminophen: N-acetylcysteine.
- Calcium channel blockers, beta-blockers: Calcium chloride, glucagon.
- Tricyclic antidepressants: Sodium bicarbonate.
- Ethylene glycol: Fomepizole.
- Iron: Deferoxamine.

103. C: Family systems theory states that members of a family have different roles and behavioral patterns, so a change in one person's behavior will affect the others in the family. The health belief model predicts health behavior with the understanding that people take a health action to avoid negative consequences if the person expects that the negative outcome can be avoided and that he/she is able to do the action. The theory of reasoned action states the actions people take voluntarily can be predicted according to their personal attitude toward the action and their perception of how others will view the action they do. The theory of planned behavior evolved from the theory of reasoned action when studies showed behavioral intention does not necessarily result in action.

104. C: A good strategy for helping a client overcome feelings of low self-esteem includes providing opportunities for the client to make decisions. Other strategies include providing companionship, listening to the client and encouraging the client to express her feelings and concerns. Positive feedback and praise should be given when earned rather than praising everything. Telling the client she has no reason to be depressed will invalidate her feelings and further lower her self-esteem. Low self-esteem is common among older adults because they have to deal with so many losses. They may become depressed, passive and dependent.

105. A: Two primary determinants of educational effectiveness include:

- Behavior modification, which involves thorough observation and measurement, identifying behavior that needs to be changed, and planning and instituting interventions to modify that behavior. Techniques include demonstrations of appropriate behavior, reinforcement, and monitoring until the new behavior is consistent.
- Compliance rates are often determined by observation, which should be done at intervals and on multiple occasions. In some cases, this may depend on self-reports or reports of others. If education is intended to improve individual health and reduce risk factors and this occurs, it is a good indication of compliance.

106. B: Motivational enhancement therapy. Other BN therapies include:

Antidepressant	Fluoxetine (Prozac®) is FDA-approved for BN.
CBT-BN	1) Psychoeducation and strategies to eat normally and avoid binging and purging. 2) Food choices expand and dysfunctional attitudes, beliefs, and avoidance behaviors are identified. 3) Maintenance and relapse-prevention strategies are covered.
Interpersonal psychotherapy	1) Interpersonal context of disorder are analyzed and problem areas identified. 2) Focus on problem areas. 3) Progress is monitored, but client is not advised to pay attention to patterns of eating or body attitudes.
Family therapy	Family assumes responsibility for ensuring the client eats a nutritious and adequate diet. Family conflicts are explored.

107. C: Schizophrenia: Personality disintegration and distortion in the perception of reality, thought processes, and social development, including delusions, withdrawal, odd behavior, hallucinations, inability to care for self, disorganized speech, catatonia, alogia (inability to speak because of mental confusion or aphasia), hearing voices, and avolition. Depression: Depressed mood, profound and constant sense of hopelessness and despair, or loss of interest in all or almost all activities. Bipolar disorder: Mood swings that may include mania, depression, or both. Narcissistic personality disorder: Heightened feeling of self-importance, persistent patterns of grandiosity, a need for admiration, disregard for other people's rights, restraint in expression of feelings, and a lack of empathy.

108. A: Kolb's model of experiential learning is based on acquiring knowledge through grasping experience and transforming that experience into knowledge through cognitive processes and perception. Experience may be transformed into knowledge through abstract conceptualizing (analyzing, thinking), observation of others, or actively experimenting. This model stresses that the individual makes choices between the concrete and the abstract, and this is reflected in learning styles:
- Diverging: Concrete experience and reflective observation
- Assimilating: Abstract conceptualization and reflective observation
- Converging: Abstract conceptualization and active experimentation
- Accommodating: Concrete experience and reflective observation

109. A: According to Piaget's theory of cognitive development, in the concrete operational stage, cause and effect is better understood and children have a good ability to understand concrete objects and the concept of conservation. Stages include:
- Sensorimotor (0–24 months): Intellect begins to develop and children acquire motor and reasoning skills, begin to use language, and prepare for more complex intellectual activities.
- Preoperational (2–7 years): Children develop a beginning concept of cause and effect along with magical thinking and egocentrism.
- Concrete operational (7–11 years): Children understand cause and effect, concrete objects, and the concept of conservation. Formal operational (11years –adult): Children/young adults develop mature though processes, ability to think abstractly, and evaluate different possibilities and outcomes.

110. B: Situational/Dispositional crises result from a response to an external stressor, such as the loss of a job, that leaves the person feeling helpless and unable to cope.

Adventitious/Social crises result from natural disasters, violent crimes, acts of terrorism, or socially disruptive acts, such as rioting, over which a person has little control. Maturational/Developmental crises occur during major life transitions, such as getting married, leaving home, or having a child. Psychopathological crises result from a preexisting psychiatric disorder, such as schizophrenia.

111. C: Chess and Thomas's temperament theory describes nine personality parameters to describe how children (≥4 weeks) respond to events. These personality traits explain the difficult child, the child who is slow to warm up to new people and circumstances, and the child who is easy to manage and adaptable. Resilience theory describes the ability of children to function in healthy ways despite adverse circumstances. Bandura's social learning theory proposes that children learn from interacting with adults and their peers and through modeling behavior. Kohlberg's theory of moral development outlines the progressive stages in which children develop a sense of morality.

112. A: "The law doesn't allow me to give out any information about patients in order to protect their privacy and safety" is accurate and appropriate. The Health Insurance Portability and Accountability Act (HIPAA) addresses the privacy of health information. Psychiatric/mental health nurses must not release any information or documentation about a patient's condition or treatment without consent. Personal information about the patient is considered protected health information (PHI), and includes any identifying or personal information about the patient, such as health history, condition, or treatments in any form, and any documentation. Failure to comply with HIPAA regulations can make a nurse liable for legal action.

113. D: RCMAS assesses anxiety in children and adolescents (6–19) with 37 yes-no questions and can be read to young children. HAS [MORE COMMON ACRONYM APPEARS TO BE "HAMA"] provides an evaluation of overall anxiety and its degree of severity for children and adults. This scale is frequently utilized in psychotropic drug evaluations. BAI is a tool for adolescents and adults that ranks 21 common symptoms related to anxiety according to the degree they have bothered the client in the previous month. BDI is a widely utilized, self-reported, multiple-choice questionnaire consisting of 21 items, which measures the degree of depression for those 17 to 80 years.

114. C: Adolescents respond well to a combination of SSRI and CBT for the treatment of depression, but SSRI use in adolescents has been associated with increased suicidal ideation, so the girl must be carefully monitored and assessed. She and her family should be educated about this possible effect and the warning signs of suicidal ideation. In some cases, adolescents may be asked to sign a no-suicide contract that clearly outlines the steps to take in the event they feel suicidal.

115. D: Targeted. Primary prevention strategies include:
- Targeted: Aimed at a select group or subgroup with perceived risk. Strategies may include encouraging physicians to intervene with brief advice, such as advising all adolescents about dangers of substance abuse.
- Universal: Aimed at the entire population; non-specific. These strategies may include mass marketing procedures, such as multimedia anti-drug campaigns aimed at the general public.
- Indicated: Aimed at individuals at high risk, such as adolescents in environments with heavy drug use.

- Secondary prevention includes efforts to prevent further drug abuse, such as Narcotics Anonymous.

116. C: Ego integrity vs despair. Erikson's stages include:

Trust vs mistrust	Birth to 1 year	Can result in mistrust or faith and optimism
Autonomy vs shame/doubt	1–3 years	Can lead to doubt and shame or self-control and willpower
Initiative vs guilt	3–6 years	Can lead to guilt or direction and purpose
Industry vs inferiority	6–12 years	Can lead to inadequacy and inferiority or competence
Identity vs role confusion	12–18 years	Can lead to role confusion or devotion and fidelity to others
Intimacy vs isolation	Young adulthood	Can lead to lack of close relationships or love/intimacy
Generativity vs stagnation	Middle age	Can lead to stagnation or caring and achievements
Ego integrity vs despair	Older adulthood	Can lead to despair (failure to accept changes of aging) or wisdom (acceptance)

117. B: Monoamine oxidase inhibitors (MAOIs) should not be taken with alcohol and non-alcoholic substitutes for beer or wine, foods high in tyramine (organ meats, cured meats, caviar, cheese products, avocados, bananas, raisins, soy, and fava beans), and products containing caffeine (tea, cola, chocolate, and coffee). MAOIs are older antidepressant medications that are used less frequently now that others are available because they have significant side effects and interactions with other medications, such as decongestants, opioids, and antidepressants.

118. A: The initial intervention for an emotional crisis reflecting psychopathology is to stay with the patient and reassure her until her panic subsides. People with borderline personality disorder (BPD) feel insecure and inherently worthless. They are often erratic and have difficulty establishing long-term relationships, although symptoms tend to lessen with age. The main feature of BPD is a persistent pattern of instability in interpersonal relationships, self-image, and emotion. Two-thirds of those diagnosed are female. Characteristics include attempts to avoid real or imagined abandonment and impulsivity in at least two areas.

119. B: Making observations is stating what is perceived, such as "I notice you are wringing your hands." Presenting reality is stating what is true or real. For example, if a patient states, "I hear someone screaming," the nurse might state, "That is an ambulance siren." Reflecting is directing the patient's thoughts, actions, or feelings back to the patient. If the patient states, "My husband says I should stop therapy," the nurse might say, "Do you think you should?" Giving recognition is acknowledging what is perceived, for example, telling the patient, "I notice that you've combed your hair and put on makeup."

120. A: Subjective notes usually quote what the client states directly: "I don't want to do this!" Objective notes record what is observed, or clinical facts: "Patient sitting with arms

folded, yawning frequently, and closing eyes." Assessment relates to the evaluation of subjective and objective notes: "Patient appears tired. He has been complaining of insomnia." Plan is based on assessment: "Administer antidepressant in the morning rather than at bedtime and schedule daily nap."

121. D: This is a mixed group.

Groups classified according to form	
Homogeneous	Members chosen on a selected basis, such as abused women
Heterogeneous	Group includes an assortment of individuals with different diagnoses, ages, genders
Mixed	Group members share some key features, such as the same diagnosis, but differ in age or gender
Closed	Group has a stable membership and excludes new members
Open	Group may vary from meeting to meeting because the members and leaders change

122. A: Once a person completes gender reassignment surgery and legally changes genders, that person is then considered the reassigned gender; thus, Mikaela is considered female, so her attraction to other females would result in her sexual orientation as lesbian. If she were attracted to males, she would be heterosexual. While she could also be classified as homosexual, this term is more commonly used for gay males, and she is no longer considered a male. She does not report a bisexual attraction to both genders.

123. D: The patient most likely at risk is the man who shot himself in the chest while alone. A suicide risk assessment should evaluate some of the following criteria: Would the individual sign a contract for safety? Is there a suicide plan? How lethal is the plan? What is the elopement risk? How often are the suicidal thoughts, and has the person attempted suicide before? High-risk findings include:
- Violent suicide attempt (knives, gunshots).
- Suicide attempt with low chance of rescue.
- Ongoing psychosis or disordered thinking.
- Ongoing severe depression and feeling of helplessness.
- History of previous suicide attempts.
- Lack of social support system.

124. C: A number of different types of outcomes data must be considered when evaluating outcomes data:
- Integrative (includes measures of mortality, longevity, and cost-effectiveness)
- Clinical (includes symptoms, diagnoses, staging of disease, and indicators of individual health)
- Physiological (includes measures of physical abnormalities, loss of function, and activities of daily living)
- Psychosocial (includes feelings, perceptions, beliefs, functional impairment, and role performance)
- Perception (includes customer perceptions, evaluations, and satisfaction)
- Organization-wide clinical (includes re-admissions, adverse reactions, and deaths)

125.D: Loose association is jumping from one topic to another with little coherence although the content is understandable. Word salad is a flow of incoherent disconnected words that do not convey meaning. Flight of ideas is speech that is excessive and rapid, with unrelated ideas: "The car is new. The dog barked all night, and the moon was out. I need some water." Evasion is avoidance of making clear statements: "I ... um ... think ... that could be ... perhaps ... right." Neologism is the creation of new words.

126. A: Akinesia is the inability to start a movement. The extrapyramidal system is a group of neural connections outside of the medulla that control movement. Extrapyramidal effects are the result of drug influence on the extrapyramidal system and also include:
- Akathisia (inability to stop movement).
- Dystonia (extreme and uncontrolled muscle contraction, torticollis, flexing, and twisting).
- Bradykinesia (slowness of movement; also characteristic of Parkinson's disease).
- Tardive dyskinesia (inability to control movement such as tics, lip smacking, and eye blinking).

127. B: NDNQI provides unit level data to help determine the quality of nursing care by comparing data with other units and national averages. The NCHS compiles all types of health information from multiple sources in order to help document health status, monitor trends, support research, and identify needs and disparities. The NDI has provided records of death since 1979, compiled from state offices of vital statistics. This information may be used by researchers for statistical purposes only. MedlinePlus is a website produced by the National Library of Medicine to provide the general public access to information about health.

128. D: The Life Safety Code® (NFPA 101) is produced by the National Fire Protection Association in order to prevent fires. The Life Safety Code® is a set of standards rather than laws or regulations, but the standards are widely followed and laws usually conform to the standards. The Life Safety Code® focuses on fire-safe construction for various types of facilities, including hospitals, and applies to new construction as well as existing structures, vehicles, and vessels. The Life Safety Code® ranks the flame spread of materials.

129. B: Gross negligence. Negligence indicates that *proper care* has not been provided, based on established standards. *Reasonable care* uses a rationale for decision-making in relation to providing care. Types of negligence include:
- Negligent conduct (indicates that an individual failed to provide reasonable care or to protect/assist another, based on standards and expertise).
- Gross negligence (willfully providing inadequate care while disregarding the safety and security of another).
- Contributory negligence (involves the injured party contributing to his/her own harm).
- Comparative negligence (attempts to determine what percentage amount of negligence is attributed to each individual involved).

130. D: Lithium is administered as a lithium salt in the form of lithium carbonate or lithium citrate. The sodium in lithium attaches more readily to sodium receptors on cells than the sodium in sodium chloride (table salt), so low sodium intake prevents adequate uptake. Additionally, excretion of lithium is associated with excretion of sodium, so hyponatremia results in decreased excretion of lithium, causing toxic levels to develop. Patients on lithium must have adequate sodium and fluid intake.

131. C: The most important consideration is the education and skills of the person to whom the task is delegated. Five rights of delegation include:

- Right task: Determine an appropriate task to delegate for a specific patient.
- Right circumstance: Consider the setting, resources, time factors, safety factors, and all other relevant information to determine the appropriateness of delegation.
- Right person: Choose the right person (by virtue of education/skills) to perform a task for the right patient.
- Right direction: Provide a clear description of the task, the purpose, any limits, and expected outcomes.
- Right supervision: Supervise, intervene as needed, and evaluate performance of the task.

132. A: Steps to conflict resolution include:

- First, allow both sides to present their side of conflict without bias, maintaining a focus on opinions rather than individuals.
- Encourage cooperation through negotiation and compromise.
- Maintain the focus, providing guidance to keep the discussions on track and avoid arguments.
- Evaluate the need for renegotiation, formal resolution process, or third party.

The best time for conflict resolution is when differences emerge but before open conflict and hardening of positions occur. The nurse must pay close attention to the people and problems involved, listen carefully, and reassure those involved that their points of view are understood.

133. D: Prealbumin (transthyretin) is most commonly monitored for acute changes in nutritional status because it has a half-life of only 2 to 3 days.

- Mild deficiency: 10–15mg/dL
- Moderate deficiency: 5–9 mg/dL
- Severe deficiency: <5 mg/dL

Prealbumin is a good measurement because it quickly decreases when nutrition is inadequate and rises quickly in response to increased protein intake. Protein intake must be adequate to maintain levels of prealbumin. Total protein and transferrin levels can be influenced by many factors. Albumin has a half-life of 18 to 20 days, so it is sensitive to long-term protein deficiencies more than short-term.

134. B: For recertification, 50% of continuing education courses must be from formally approved providers while the other 50% may include in-service hours, workshops, and other training provided by the place of employment. Independent study or Internet study is acceptable. Additionally, 51% of the hours must be directly related to psychiatric/mental health nursing. Certification lasts for 5 years. Other requirements of recertification include 1000 hours of practice in the area of certification in the 5 years preceding recertification.

135. A: Cost-benefit analysis uses average cost of an event and the cost of intervention to demonstrate savings. Cost-effective analysis measures the effectiveness of an intervention rather than the monetary savings. Efficacy studies may compare a series of cost-benefit analyses to determine the intervention with the best cost benefit. They may also be used for

process or product evaluation. Cost-utility analysis is essentially a sub-type of cost-effective analysis, but it is more complex and the results are more difficult to quantify and use to justify expense because cost-utility analysis measures benefit to society in general, such as decreasing teen pregnancy.

136. B: According to the American Geriatrics Society Guideline for the Prevention of Falls in Older Persons, if a patient has one fall, the patient should be assessed for gait and balance, including the get-up-and-go test in which the patient stands up from a chair without using arms to assist, walks across the room, and returns. If the patient is steady, no further assessment is needed. If the patient demonstrates unsteadiness, further assessment to determine the cause is necessary.

137. C: Patient report is the most important criterion for determining the degree of a patient's pain. People may perceive and express pain very differently, so unless drug-seeking or attention-seeking behavior can be established, the psychiatric/mental health nurse should accept the patient's degree of pain as reported. Some cultures encourage outward expressions of pain while others do not. Various pain scales may be used, depending on the age and cognitive ability of the patient. The most commonly used scale for adolescents and adults is the one-to-ten scale.

138. A: AIMS is an assessment tool to evaluate tardive dyskinesia in those taking antipsychotic medications. The CAGE tool is used as a quick assessment tool to determine if people are drinking excessively or are problem drinkers. MMSE is used to assess cognition in those with evidence of dementia or short-term memory loss associated with Alzheimer's disease. CAM is used to assess the development of delirium and is intended primarily for those without psychiatric training.

139. D: The psychiatric/mental health nurse engaged as a consultation liaison primarily is expected to assess psychiatric disorders and emotional needs of medical, surgical, and obstetric patients. The nurse may assess dementia, confusion, depression, and delirium. Patients are seen upon request of the medical staff primarily responsible for the patient's care, usually when questions about the patient's mental status or ability to make informed decisions arise. In some cases, assessment for suicide or homicide risk or substance abuse may be indicated.

140. A: The initial presentation should include a summary of the data. A PowerPoint® or similar presentation is excellent because the information can be presented in graphs or charts. A presenter should always avoid reading a report verbatim, as this is often boring and hard to follow. Raw data should be available for those who are interested, but beginning with raw data may be confusing. Discussions are good following the report, but the purpose is to dispense information rather than determine what information people want.

141. C: "Anxiety" is an actual diagnosis determined by clinical judgment based on history, assessment, signs, and symptoms. "Risk for acute confusion" is an example of a risk diagnosis associated with risk factors and response to condition. "Readiness for enhanced relationship" is an example of a health promotion diagnosis based on the motivation of a patient or family members to improve health and functioning. "Post-trauma syndrome" is an example of a syndrome diagnosis based on a group of nursing diagnoses that require similar treatment.

142. D: For most drugs, including methamphetamines, testing hair provides information for the longest period. Urine tests are positive for methamphetamines for 3 to 5 days, and both blood and oral fluids for only 1 to 3 days, while hair testing is positive for up to 90 days. The length of time for positive findings in urine, blood, and oral fluids varies widely depending on the drug. However, with the exception of alcohol, which is positive in the hair only for up to 2 days, most drugs are detectable in hair for up to 90 days.

143. B: Children ages 9 to 17 should be restrained and/or secluded no longer than 2 hours while children <9 should only be restrained and/or secluded for a maximum of 1 hour. Restraints should be used only as a last resort in cases where the child and/or others are threatened, and the patient should be released as soon as it is safe to do so. Children must be frequently monitored during the duration of restraint and seclusion, and pressure and unsafe holds should not be applied to children in restraints.

144. B: Left hemisphere strokes are characterized by these symptoms. Right hemisphere strokes result in left paralysis or paresis and a left visual field deficit. Fine motor skills may be impacted, resulting in trouble dressing or handling tools. People may become impulsive, depressed, and exhibit poor judgment. They often deny impairment, and may have short-term memory loss, but language remains intact. Brain stem strokes may involve motor and/or sensory impairment and respiratory and cardiac abnormalities. Cerebellar strokes may result in ataxia, nausea and vomiting, headaches, and dizziness or vertigo.

145. C: While all of these are important, patients who are homeless require further assistance with discharge, as compliance with treatment and follow-up appointments is poor in the homeless population. Interventions that are most important include:
- Lists of safe shelters and places they can go to bathe, eat, and get mail.
- Assistance in applying for welfare assistance or Social Security.

Discharge planning should begin on admission and must be a joint effort so that the transfer and discharge documents provide the information that the individual needs.

146. A: An increase in the total white blood cell (WBC) count accompanied by a shift to the left, or increase in bands (immature neutrophils) and neutrophils, usually indicates an acute bacterial infection. Normal WBC counts may range from approximately 5,000 to 10,000, but can increase rapidly with acute infection, such as appendicitis, as the bone marrow produces more neutrophils to combat the infection. Because cells are produced rapidly, increased numbers of immature cells (bands) are also released into the blood stream.

147. C: The AACAP has established 3 criteria for the use of ECT in adolescents:
- They must have completed at least 2 drug trials combined with other therapy without improvement in symptoms.
- Diagnoses may include major depression/mania with or without associated psychotic symptoms, schizophrenia (in some instances), or schizoaffective disorders. (ECT is less successful as treatment of psychotic disorders than mood disorders.)
- Symptoms are severe, disabling, and may be life-threatening.

148. D: The most immediate goal is to manage the patient's symptoms with appropriate medications and for the patient to take only prescribed medications rather than self-medicating with cocaine and alcohol. Patients with dual diagnoses can present challenges

because they cannot abstain from all medications if their symptoms are to be controlled. Once they are properly medicated, they can begin to interact with others, express feeling, and develop plans for activities. When stabilized, they can begin to work on social skills and participate in alcohol/drug-free activities.

149. B: Tracer methodology looks at the continuum of care a patient receives from admission to post-discharge. A patient is selected to be "traced" and the medical record serves as a guide. Tracer methodology uses the experience of this patient to evaluate the processes in place through documents and interviews. Root cause analysis (RCA) is a retrospective attempt to determine the cause of an event, often a sentinel event such as an unexpected death, or a cluster of events. RCA involves interviews, observations, and review of medical records. Family and staff surveys may provide helpful but less detailed information.

150. D: In most cases, careful observation of patients with Alzheimer's disease can help to determine what triggers agitation or outbursts so the triggers can be eliminated. When Alzheimer's patients have too much input or feel overwhelmed, they react negatively. Isolating the patient is rarely the answer and decreases social interaction. Making choices can be confusing and difficult, so asking patients to choose may increase agitation. Antipsychotic medications are generally contraindicated for Alzheimer's patients and do not attend to the underlying problem.